Living with HIV in Post-Crisis Times

Anthropology of Well-Being

Individual, Community, Society

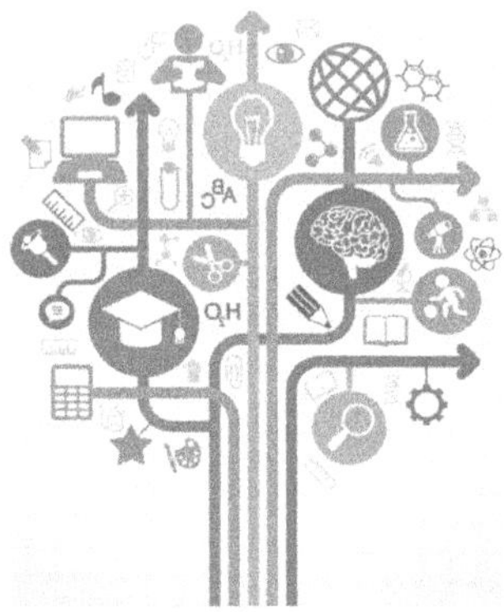

***Series Editor*:** Ben G. Blount, PhD (SocioEcological Informatics)

Mission Statement

Well-being is central and important in people's daily lives and life history. This book series brings about understanding of what the complex concepts of well-being include. The concepts of quality of life, life satisfaction, and happiness will be explored and viewed at the individual level, the community level, and the level of society. The series encourages and promotes research into the concept of well-being, how it appears to be defined culturally, and how it is utilized across levels and across different social, economic, and ethnic groups. Understandings of how well-being promotes stability and resilience will also be critical to advances in understanding, as well as how well-being can be implemented as a goal in resisting vulnerabilities and in adaptation. Series books include monographs and edited collections by a range of academics, from rising scholars to experts in relevant fields.

Recent Titles in the Series

Living with HIV in Post-Crisis Times: Beyond the Endgame, edited by David A. B. Murray

Diversity and Cultural Competence in the Health Sector: Ebola-Affected Countries in West Africa, by Mohamed Kanu, Elizabeth A. Williams, Charles Williams, and Regina Bash-Taqi

Everyday Food Practices: Commercialisation and Consumption in the Periphery of the Global North, by Tarunna Sebastian

No Perfect Birth: Trauma and Obstetric Care in the Rural United States, by Kristin Haltinner

Love and Its Entanglements among the Enxet of Paraguay: Social and Kinship Relations within a Market Economy, by Stephen Kidd

Living with HIV in Post-Crisis Times

Beyond the Endgame

Edited by
David A. B. Murray

LEXINGTON BOOKS
Lanham • Boulder • New York • London

Published by Lexington Books
An imprint of The Rowman & Littlefield Publishing Group, Inc.
4501 Forbes Boulevard, Suite 200, Lanham, Maryland 20706
www.rowman.com

86-90 Paul Street, London EC2A 4NE

British Library Cataloguing in Publication Information Available

Library of Congress Cataloging-in-Publication Data

Names: Murray, David A. B., 1962- editor.
Title: Living with HIV in post-crisis times : beyond the endgame / edited by David A.B. Murray.
Description: Lanham : Lexington Books, [2021] | Series: Anthropology of well-being: individual, community, society | Includes bibliographical references and index.
Identifiers: LCCN 2021025140 (print) | LCCN 2021025141 (ebook) | ISBN 9781666901481 (cloth) | ISBN 9781666901498 (epub)
Subjects: LCSH: AIDS (Disease) | HIV (Viruses) | AIDS (Disease)—Social aspects.
Classification: LCC RC607.A26 .L59 2021 (print) | LCC RC607.A26 (ebook) | DDC 616.97/92—dc23
LC record available at https://lccn.loc.gov/2021025140
LC ebook record available at https://lccn.loc.gov/2021025141

Contents

Acknowledgments

The genesis of this book was a double panel presentation at the 2019 American Anthropological Association Annual Meetings in Vancouver, Canada. Kasey Beduhn from Lexington Books contacted me prior to the meetings and provided encouragement for this collection of papers to be developed and expanded into an edited book. This project was supported through Development and Insight Grants from the Social Sciences and Humanities Research Council of Canada. A deep thank-you to Kasey Beduhn and the staff at Lexington Books for their ongoing support throughout all stages of the publication process. I would also like to thank all the contributors to this book for their time, work, and constructive feedback in developing their papers into a cohesive set of chapters reflecting the key objectives and themes that generated this book. I would like to dedicate this book to all people living with HIV (approximately 38 million people across the globe were living with HIV/AIDS in 2019 according to UNAIDS) many of whom continue to face ongoing daily struggles for survival generated through longstanding global political and economic inequities.

Introduction

David A. B. Murray

Over the past few years, and now on the cusp of its fifth decade as a "global pandemic," HIV/AIDS (human immunodeficiency virus/acquired immunodeficiency syndrome) has mostly disappeared from North American mainstream news coverage and the public sphere. When it is mentioned, we tend to see optimistic headlines like "End to AIDS in sight as huge study finds drugs stop HIV transmission" (Boseley and Devline 2019) or "The end of the HIV crisis is within our grasp" (Rourke and Flanagan 2020; see also McKinley 2019). Global public health organizations like the United Nations Program on HIV/AIDS (UNAIDS) issue statements that HIV/AIDS is now a manageable, chronic illness, thanks to advances in treatment medications that have caused a substantial global drop in HIV transmission rates and deaths from AIDS,[1] leading these organizations to declare that the AIDS epidemic can be ended by 2030.[2] In these "end of crisis" headlines, the narrative arc of HIV/AIDS has shifted from one of tragedy, suffering, and death to one of hope, optimism, and life. Now, in many parts of the world, people living with HIV (PLHIV) are told not only that they will not die from AIDS-related complications but that they will be able to lead "near normal" lifespans as long as they adhere to a daily regimen of medication known as antiretroviral therapy (ART) for the rest of their lives. More recently, PLHIV have been informed that if they adhere to their daily ART regimen, they cannot transmit the virus to anyone: Biomedical research has proven that people with HIV who achieve and maintain an undetectable viral load—the amount of HIV in the blood—by taking ART daily as prescribed cannot sexually transmit the virus to others[3] (Public Health Agency of Canada 2017), which further contributes to the message that HIV can be managed, if not eradicated, through treatment as prevention (Cohen 2011; Vernooij et al. 2016) and that PLHIV are now able to lead "near normal" lives with little fear and uncertainty about their own health status and its impact on others, thus experiencing less stigma attached to their HIV+ (positive) status. In order to facilitate a "return" to "near normal" life, PLHIV are encouraged by public health organizations and/or HIV/AIDS support services to embrace "positive living," a "disease-based identity movement" premised upon a set of practices and values that contribute toward improving and maintaining physical health, making changes in attitude and self-perception, and demonstrating levels of self-sufficiency, responsibility, and expressed concern about long-term self-care (Benton, Sangaramoorthy and Kalofonos 2017:455).

However, as numerous HIV researchers and activists have pointed out, "end of AIDS crisis," and "HIV as a chronic, manageable illness" narratives, along with "positive living" therapeutic rubrics, are highly contested and carry within them problematic biomedical assumptions about health, data, time, personhood, and sociality that do not acknowledge the fluidity and flexibility of disease conditions over the life course (Colvin 2011, Manderson and Smith Morris 2010, Sangaramoorthy 2018), nor do they question where, how, why, and for whom optimistic narratives about HIV's normalization, management, and future may actually contribute to or worsen a state of crisis (Benton et al. 2017). As a number of this book's authors point out, "end of crisis" and "HIV as chronic illness" narratives do not, for the most part, address the impact of stagnant or decreasing funding of the global HIV/AIDS response,[4] and/or gloss over significant local, national, and global differences and disparities in the management and control of the pandemic, and their effects on HIV+ populations. For example, as Benton et al. observe, management of PLHIV populations through "positive living" rubrics, particularly those in the Global South and marginalized Global North communities, is often shaped by a history of Western technoscientific intervention that has influenced assumptions about difference, modernity, and the future, producing a particular image of how to be a good, healthy, and productive HIV+ person while pathologizing anyone who does not ascribe to this particular set of practices and affirmations, thus reinforcing colonial tropes of racialized, backward, and irrational subjects. Positive living programs in the Global South and marginalized Global North communities are thus constructed through the threat of the "failed subject," generated in part through comparisons to the "progressive" model of the HIV/AIDS industry of the Global North (Benton et al. 2017, Nguyen 2005, Patton 2002). The HIV/AIDS industry is "a complex assemblage of state, civil society and corporate actors and . . . forms of biomedical, pharmaceutical, behavioural, epidemiological . . . expertise, discourse, policy and technology" (located primarily in the Global North) that are drawn on to know and respond to HIV/AIDS as a governable problem with "evidence"-based solutions that will soon lead to its eradication (Mykhalovskiy and Namaste

2019:9). However, the HIV/AIDS industry's Global North-centric, managerial, data-driven, and biotechnological approach to eradicating the threat of HIV does not, for the most part, attend to structural inequities on various scales, nor does it adequately locate HIV/AIDS in specific social, economic, and political contexts in order to better understand localized effects and responses (Mykhalovskiy and Namaste 2019).

Given these recent developments in and critiques of global discourses about "the end of HIV/AIDS," (bio)technological knowledge about and (re) classification of HIV/AIDS as a "chronic, manageable" disease, and models of governance and management of PLHIV populations through "positive living," the authors in this book were invited to submit papers that address three interrelated themes and attendant questions arising from this current historical moment of the HIV/AIDS pandemic, utilizing conceptual frameworks and methods which anchor these themes and questions in specific social, economic, and political contexts in order to explore localized effects and responses:

1) Challenging "end of crisis" narratives: How are "end of the HIV/AIDS crisis" discourses political tools as much as public health goals, and how do they amplify rifts and inequalities in the global HIV/AIDS response? How are diverse communities of PLHIV (and the organizations supporting them) mediating notions of difference, self, and health through "end of crisis" narratives alongside an increasing global political economy of metrics that circumscribes conditions of possibility for civil society entities such as community-based organizations? How are PLHIV and their support organizations navigating stagnant or decreasing public interest and local, national, and global funding for the HIV response?
2) Reflecting on the meanings and effects of HIV's reclassification as a chronic illness: If HIV is now considered to be a "chronic" illness (as long as PLHIV have access to and regularly take ART medications), what are the logics and effects of HIV chronicity? How are conceptions of time embedded in public health programs directed at HIV+ people who are now living with a "chronic" illness (Benton et al. 2017)? While biotechnical strategies may now address and control the physiological symptoms of HIV/AIDS, they may not necessarily address the psychological or social ones. Therefore, the chronicity of HIV/AIDS is not (only) a medical fact but (also) a technological, political, and economic one (Smith Morris in Sangaramoorthy 2018). Keeping this expanded definition of HIV chronicity in mind, how does the reclassification of "HIV as a chronic illness" impact the funding and organization of public health infrastructures, HIV/AIDS support services, and their management of PLHIV populations? How does this chronic status

effect PLHIV experiences of stigma and disclosure? Does it contribute toward the amelioration of economic and social challenges experienced by PLHIV?

3) Analyzing "positive living" rubrics: Positive living is an evolving set of moral, physical, and social therapeutic practices developed since the advent of antiretroviral therapies (Benton et al. 2017). How are positive living programs/practices (re)formed in the "end of crisis" era and/or as HIV/AIDS is increasingly defined as a chronic and manageable illness? How does "positive living" with a chronic illness infer particular notions of time, difference, health, and the self in past, present, and future therapeutic frameworks? How do differentially positioned PLHIV communities (dis)engage with "positive living" programs and (re)define positive living for themselves?

In critically examining these three themes reflecting a particular historical moment in the global HIV/AIDS response, the contributors to this book challenge the Global North-centric, biomedical, metrics-driven, and managerial frameworks that dominate so much of the HIV/AIDS industry today. Utilizing primarily ethnographic methods, these chapters explore the contemporary governance and management of HIV/AIDS and PLHIV communities in different locations around the globe (India, South Africa, Uganda, West Africa,[5] Canada, Jamaica, Japan, and Egypt) and reveal how diverse communities of PLHIV and/or organizations supporting them navigate an array of physical, social, political, and economic challenges in so-called "post-crisis" times. In doing so, they make an important contribution to critical social science research on HIV/AIDS.

CRITICAL SOCIAL SCIENCE RESEARCH ON HIV/AIDS

Critical social science research on HIV/AIDS has made important interventions into hegemonic biomedical and epidemiological frameworks since the early years of the pandemic, demonstrating how the specificities and contingencies of transnational forces, structural violence, political economy, and asymmetric power relations of race, class, gender, and sexuality shape the conditions of HIV risk and vulnerability (Benton et al. 2017; Butt 2005; Comaroff 2007; Farmer 2006 [1992], 2001 [1991], 2003; Herdt 1987; Jolivette 2016; MacQueen 1994; McGrath et al. 2014; Moyer 2015; Patton 1990, 2002; Singer et al. 1990; Sangaramoorthy 2018; Smith 2014; Sobo 1999; Treichler 1999; Wardlow 2008; Yingling 1997). That is, "people are differentially exposed to HIV on the basis of their social locations in ways that mirror exposure and vulnerability to damaging structures of inequality, requiring approaches that account for the epidemic's intersectional inequalities" (Watkins-Hayes 2014, 433).

Critical social science research has also queried how responses to HIV/AIDS engender new forms of life (subjectivities, affects, and conduct) as well as potentially constituting new communities, activisms, institutions, and publics (e.g., Benton 2015; Boellstorff 2009, 2011; Lorway 2017; Pigg 2001). As the global rollout of ART transformed the status of HIV/AIDS from terminal to chronic, giving rise to what has been called "the age of treatment" (Moyer 2015), researchers observed the development of "therapeutic citizenship," the network of state and nongovernmental organizations involved in the definition and maintenance of healthy populations as moral and ethical projects that develop techniques to control, manage, and assess bodies (Nguyen 2010; see also Nguyen et al. 2011, and Whyte's [2014] discussion of "clientship"). Therapeutic citizenship, which incorporates "positive living" rubrics, helps to elucidate the ways in which some PLHIV are named, normalized, and "responsibilized" as acceptable citizens through public health models in the age of treatment, while others are vilified as "failed subjects" and/or deemed not worthy of outreach, treatment, and support (Biehl 2007; Colvin et al. 2010; Igonya and Moyer 2013). Furthermore, as noted by Benton et al., the transformation of the biomedical paradigm of HIV/AIDS from terminal to chronic, resulting in new forms of therapeutic citizenship like positive living, has reorganized biomedical temporal frameworks which define and mediate notions of difference, health, and the self in different sociocultural contexts (2017).

With a shift from an emphasis on survival to long-term living with the virus, research in the age of treatment has focused not only on new forms of governance and management of PLHIV but also on life projects of those on treatment, including the desire to have children and return to work (Smith and Mbakwem 2010; Hirsch et al. 2009; Seeley 2014), issues of dignity and privacy (Moyer 2012; Seeley 2014), the use of alternative therapies (Kalofonos 2010), shifts in family-based care arrangements (de Klerk 2011), and sexual activities (Moyer 2015). However, Mykhalovskiy and Rosengarten (2009) and Mykhalovskiy and Namaste (2019) have observed an overall decrease in theoretical and critical social inquiry into HIV/AIDS as the pandemic entered its third and fourth decades, and I would argue not much has changed as we enter its fifth decade: The lack of sustained critical social science research into (1) the organization and transformation of the management and treatment of PLHIV; (2) changing relationships between global HIV/AIDS funding organizations, regional/state public health systems, and local HIV/AIDS service organizations; and (3) new biomedical knowledge and discourses about HIV/AIDS prevention, transmission, and treatment, means that new forms of knowledge about HIV/AIDS continue to emanate primarily (and problematically) from clinical, epidemiological, and positivist science perspectives.

There are, however, important exceptions to this trend: Over the past decade there continues to have been a small, but steady output of ethnographic research unpacking the complex realities of HIV/AIDS prevention and treatment programs, ongoing multiple challenges for differentially positioned PLHIV communities around the globe, and creative activism emanating from those communities, sometimes resulting in improved outcomes (Benton 2015, Black 2019, Heckert 2018, Kenworthy 2017, Marten 2020, O'Daniel 2016, Reed 2018, Sangaramoorthy 2014, Smith 2014, Whyte 2014). In addition, Mykhalovskiy and Namaste (2019) provide a collection of social science perspectives that challenge contemporary mainstream biomedical approaches to the HIV/AIDS epidemic through a range of topics including HIV criminalization, HIV disclosure, frontline community work, and biomedical prevention campaigns in North America. Kerrigan and Barrington's edited volume (2018) offers a critical analysis of the structural dynamics of HIV risk and responses among populations at heightened vulnerability, with chapters presenting grassroots initiatives that have led both to positive social change and improved HIV outcomes. Similarly, Lorway (2017) comparatively examines how HIV activism in three locations (Canada, India, and Kenya) figures into the possibility of more democratized collaborations between affected communities, scientists, and policy makers. These important ethnographic and critical social science interventions provide comparative, in-depth insights into the complex local contexts of HIV treatment and prevention programs and PLHIV experiences, powerfully underscoring the long-standing critical social science claim that intersecting sociocultural, political, and economic structures and relations of inequality are foundational to understanding, controlling, and ending the HIV/AIDS (indeed, any viral) pandemic.

CHALLENGING THE NARRATIVES: KEY FINDINGS OF THIS BOOK

This book is located firmly within the field of critical social science research on HIV/AIDS, employing many of the important theoretical and methodological insights noted above. However, this collection of ethnographic investigations into the lives of diverse groups of PLHIV around the globe, and the local, regional, and global infrastructures dedicated to their health and well-being, is the first book to provide a global comparative focus that reveals what has changed (and what has not) during the fourth decade of the pandemic (approximately 2010–2020). Building on the legacy of decades of critical social science research on HIV/AIDS, this book's contributors focus on the governance, management, and/or experiences of HIV+ lives, developing insights that extend beyond biomedical, metrics-based assessments of "vulnerable," "at-risk," and/or "key" populations, and providing more nuanced and holistic forms of analysis that not only reveal the multiple and diverse challenges and successes of differentially positioned PLHIV individuals, organizations, and communities but also reframe thinking on the management of a long-term epidemic on local, national, and global scales.

More specifically, this edited book provides ethnographically informed examinations of how HIV+ communities and organizations dedicated to maintaining the health and well-being of these communities in different locations around the world are navigating the material, social, and economic consequences of "end of crisis," "HIV as a chronic disease," and "HIV normalization" discourses in a climate of decreasing financial, political, and popular support, alongside new and ongoing therapeutic interventions that include (but are not limited to) "positive living" rubrics.

Collectively, they reveal a number of important insights about the HIV/AIDS pandemic as it enters its fifth decade: First, they demonstrate that not only is the HIV/AIDS crisis not over or about to end in many parts of the world but that it is actually becoming more acute for many communities in multiple locations, due in no small part to the political, economic, and social effects of "end of crisis" narratives. As Benton observes in her review of the book's chapters, "end of HIV/AIDS crisis" narratives can turn into a political tool as much as an ethical ideal or public health goalpost, producing new forms of stigma and discrimination for particular categories of PLHIV. Space-time relations, via a discourse of the "end of AIDS," become compressed or confused with each other, amplifying rifts and inequalities in many of the places discussed in this book. The political dimensions and effects of end of crisis narratives can be seen in Hassan's chapter analyzing the post-2011 revolution Egyptian government's claim to have developed a device that "cures" HIV, and the experiences of some Egyptian PLHIV who were recruited to test the device. Hassan's analysis reveals how this (completely false) claim illustrates the ways in which global health "end of AIDS crisis" aspirations may have unintended effects by increasing competition between variously positioned states and their public health infrastructures in order be the first to successfully "end AIDS," in which PLHIV become pawns in international political games. Murray's chapter illustrates a different relationship to "end of crisis" narratives, through an exploration of how a group of older gay men in Toronto, Canada, who have been living with HIV for decades, view end of AIDS narratives with suspicion and resentment: For most of this group's members, who are in their 60s and older, the physical, social, and political challenges of an HIV+ status have not receded, but rather transformed over time: Based on long-term experiences and challenges of living with HIV, they are suspicious of the claim that biomedical and pharmaceutical interventions will end the crisis, and they are resentful for the ways in which these narratives invisibilize their ongoing health issues and experiences of discrimination in the Canadian public health system, public spaces, and their own gay community.

Second, this book's chapters reveal the political and moral complexity of the proclamation that HIV is now a "chronic" illness, a biomedical reframing based on the effectiveness and availability of ART that has transformed the virus's effect from terminal to chronic, and thus (at least in theory) transformed experiences and perceptions of bodies that live with the virus, while also contributing to the "end of crisis" narratives as noted above. However, this book's authors show that a change in biomedical status (from terminal to chronic) does not necessarily translate to a change in the quality of life, nor the complexity of challenges of living with HIV: Ordóñez's chapter examines the struggle in the South African public health system over how to manage a "chronic" illness, with Western medicine prioritized as the primary treatment framework, and "Traditional African Medicine," a set of therapeutic practices accessed by mostly Black South African PLHIV, only partially acknowledged as a meaningful intervention. Saria's chapter illustrates how in India, for *hijras* (an Indian term which roughly translates to transgender) and PLHIV living in poverty, ARTs are not easily accessed due to discriminatory treatment in clinics and/or difficulties in finding work which results in constant migration; these forms of discrimination or economic difficulties speak to other forms of "chronicity," that is, ongoing cycles of prejudice and/or poverty that form a continuous crisis of survival which compounds the challenges of living with HIV. Lorway's concluding chapter to this book argues that in the "end of crisis" era of HIV chronicity, there has been no significant change in the temporal, political, and economic effects of the global health system of reporting lines, metrics, or project time on PLHIV lives and support services for PLHIV. In other words, we are still witnessing "a biopolitical regime that reduces bodies to targets of pathogenic containment." Nevertheless, as Lorway notes, we must also recognize that HIV chronicity produces new forms of intimacy and flourishment, and potentially new forms of PLHIV organization and resistance. Together, these chapters very much support Sangaramoorthy's proposal for "a reorientation of (the) logic of (HIV) chronicity to one that regards HIV as a continual crisis as it is lived and experienced for many around the world" (2018, 3).

Third, this book illustrates that while the transformation of HIV from terminal to chronic has resulted in claims of the "normalization of HIV/

AIDS," the reality for many PLHIV is anything but normal. In other words, the assumption that the widespread availability of ART, which effectively controls the spread of the virus within the body, would therefore lead to "near normal" lifespans and a return to "normal" everyday life for all PLHIV, has proven to be deeply problematic, as evidenced by many of the chapters in this book: From Runestad's examination of how Japanese HIV+ men strive to become "productive" Japanese citizens in the face of ongoing discriminatory beliefs that AIDS equals death, to Walsh Lang's observations on how a Ugandan clinic reinforces HIV/AIDS stigma in its rehabilitative therapies for HIV+ children by not telling some of them their positive status, to Schensul's chapter focusing on how ongoing perceptions of stigma and stress contribute toward higher levels of alcoholism among working-class HIV+ men in Mumbai, we repeatedly witness evidence demonstrating that the availability and/or daily intake of ART does not automatically translate to the maintenance or resumption of a "normal" life. In fact, all of the chapters demonstrate, in one way or another, that after more than 25 years since the advent of ART, there continue to be economic, political, and social inequities intersecting with an HIV+ status that contribute to ongoing or new physical and mental health issues for PLHIV.

These contributions thus underscore the well-established, but still under-acknowledged, argument that the HIV/AIDS response cannot be organized solely through biomedical, data-driven interventions: intersecting political, economic, and social structures of inequality operating on multiple scales (local, regional, and global) impact all dimensions of the HIV/AIDS response, from identifying "at-risk" populations, to addressing stigma and discrimination, to developing effective treatment protocols for PLHIV. Poverty (Schensul, Saria, Hassan, Thiongane, and Graham), race (Jolly and Ordóñez), age (Murray and Walsh Lang), gender (Runestad, Schensul, and Jolly), and sexuality (Saria and Murray) represent just some of the intersecting structures of inequality that impact or augment the challenges of an HIV-positive status, such that, even if ARTs can be accessed and consumed, there is no return to a "normal" life for many PLHIV.

Fourth, and finally, keeping in mind the impact of intersecting structural inequalities as noted above, these chapters collectively challenge assumptions of "positive living" as a uniform policy, therapeutic rubric, or aspirational identity, while simultaneously demonstrating its powerful governing effects on differentially positioned PLHIV populations (Benton et al. 2017). For example, while some positive living rubrics emphasize the benefits of disclosing one's status in order to overcome fear and shame (Murray 2020), others emphasize secrecy or simply do not inform people that they are HIV-positive due to their perceived inability—based on age (Walsh Lang) or economic status (Saria)—to be able to handle the impact of the diagnosis. Thiongane and Graham's chapter reveals another important dimension of "positive living" through their examination of PLHIV recruitment for Ebola (another epidemic generating virus) vaccine trials: Trial recruitment staff in different locations developed different biometric benchmarks to determine who is "positively healthy" enough to qualify for the trial, revealing that even within the biomedical domain, there is no agreed-upon definition of what it means to be "healthy" and HIV positive. Other contributors, such as Jolly and Runestad, illustrate ethico-moral orientations of positive living that challenge standard public health interventions, as they are generated through PLHIV experiences beyond the clinic: Jolly's examination of a grassroots organization by and for poor and working-class HIV+ Jamaican women reveals a different ontology of positive living, encouraging and supporting networks of care, mentorship, and community building. Runestad's discussion of how Japanese men living with HIV navigate Japanese gendered cultural norms of masculinity demonstrates how positive living is not only determined through biomedical rubrics and interventions but also through broader sociocultural norms, which in this case, emphasize certain key activities or life benchmarks in order to be viewed as a productive, respectable Japanese (male) citizen. Together, these chapters illustrate that there are significant gaps between "positive living" therapeutic frameworks developed in and through public health systems and everyday experiences of living as an HIV+ person, revealing some of the shortcomings of rehabilitative therapies that do not acknowledge the contextual political, sociocultural, and economic complexities of target PLHIV populations, and the strengths of those that do.

While this book does not, by a long shot, address many locations and dimensions of a global viral epidemic now spanning four decades, our hope is that it sheds light on variations, continuities, and changes in the management and lived experience of a unique disease that has had a massive impact on local, national, and global health structures and diverse communities around the world. We hope these chapters convey the uneven effects of a 40-year-old pandemic on differentially positioned PLHIV and provide analytical frameworks that help us to better understand why, in many parts of the world, the HIV crisis is not over, and why biomedical, data-driven, technocratic interventions are not, in and of themselves, enough. Collectively, these chapters powerfully reinforce arguments for the importance of critical social science interventions that contribute not only to more holistic, nuanced, and multifaceted understandings of HIV/AIDS interventions as we enter the fifth decade of the pandemic but also toward better understandings of and responses to other new and potential pandemics as well.

CHAPTER ORGANIZATION

Part I: Fantastic Conceits and How to Mind Them: Managing PLHIV in "Post-Crisis" Times: The chapters in this section focus on the practical, moral, and political dimensions of representing, governing, and managing PLHIV at various scales, from local support organizations to national health care systems. The chapters in this section also examine continuities and changes in the ways that HIV is framed and managed as a biomedical, economic, social, and political "problem" as it transitions from a "terminal" to "chronic" biomedical status, with a particular focus on the impact of these (re)framings on PLHIV.

Chapter 1 looks at how sexuality, gender, and poverty intersect to make "positive living" an impossibility for poor and migrant PLHIV in India. Saria examines how, over the long durée of the epidemic, the Indian public health infrastructure continues to adversely impact the majority of PLHIV via (1) the problematic distribution of ART in India and problematic organization of the Indian public health care system; (2) the ways in which some doctors interpret their patients' ART noncompliance as an inability to live with an HIV+ diagnosis, revealing the state's "staged fantasy" of HIV, which includes discriminatory assumptions about those who are poor and HIV+; and (3) due to these structural problems and discriminatory assumptions, ARTs are not easily or regularly accessed by marginalized groups like hijras and the urban and/or migrant poor.

Chapter 2 focuses on an announcement by the Egyptian Armed Forces in 2014 that they had discovered devices that detect and cure HIV and AIDS. Hassan analyzes how and why the Egyptian government circulated these announcements, and how Egyptian PLHIV responded to them. Hassan provides insight into the experiences of Egyptian PLHIV as they encounter, navigate, and resist biomedical authorities (and their HIV cure devices and clinical trials) in the context of postrevolutionary Egypt, and thus also provides important insights on the governmentality of HIV in unstable times (i.e., when the state is in political disarray, or trying to establish stability after a period of political upheaval), and the ways in which PLHIV are enmeshed in these temporal politics. Hassan demonstrates the politicized ways in which "fragile" HIV+ bodies are taken up by a chaotic and unstable "body politic" (in this case, a postrevolutionary Egyptian military government) as a means to legitimize the state's authority through its claims to be able to cure HIV.

Chapter 3 provides another perspective on the governing and management of PLHIV, through its focus on a Ugandan NGO that supports children living with HIV. This chapter provides important insights into the complexities and contextualities of disclosure and responsibility through its focus on the ways in which NGO staff teach the children about their medication and how to talk or not talk about illness, as in some cases, the decision is made not to inform a child of their HIV+ status in order to "protect" them from assumed psychological hardships associated with living with HIV. Walsh Lang's investigation reveals tensions between children's vulnerability, responsibility and agency, sustainable development paradigms and patronage networks of interdependence, and the biomedical and social meanings of health.

Drawing on a decade of collaborative anthropological and biomedical research on the sociocultural aspects of HIV treatment in South Africa, chapter 4 addresses the broader trends and challenges of implementing ART through a struggling public health system which exists alongside alternative, complementary, or traditional medicinal and health practices. This chapter develops important arguments about the limits of long-term Western biomedical HIV interventions among poor Black South Africans and Western medicine's problematic relationship with alternative forms of therapy, support, treatment used by traditional African medical practitioners for mostly poor, Black South African PLHIV. Ordóñez analyzes attempts to integrate the two systems, and in so doing, outlines the potential for (and challenges to) new forms of governance of and support for South African PLHIV.

Chapter 5 provides a unique perspective on the management of PLHIV populations through its focus on the impact of living in environments with multiple viruses and/or ongoing viral epidemics: Thiongane and Graham examine the biomedical, temporal, and political convergence of HIV and Ebola for PLHIV who are volunteering for an Ebola vaccine clinical trial taking place in multiple Canadian and West African locations. This examination of "dueling viruses" (and their attendant treatment and prevention protocols and technologies) reveals similarities and differences in the global health apparatus, the organization of health interventions related to viral epidemics, and their impact on targeted populations. More specifically, Thiongane and Graham demonstrate how the Ebola vaccine trial staff compete among each other in order to meet recruitment benchmarks and develop diverse and changing definitions to determine which PLHIV are healthy enough for the trials, revealing the nebulous dimensions of biomedical definitions of chronic illness.

Part II: Always Never Normal: Positive Living in "Post-Crisis" Times: This section's chapters examine how differentially positioned PLHIV navigate everyday living in various locations around the globe at a historical moment when HIV has receded from the public gaze and no longer circulates as a priority health concern with the same level of intensity in public spheres like media, the state, and/or the biomedical apparatus.

Chapter 6 examines how PLHIV or yōseisha (the literal translation of which is "positive person") in Japan have been actively fighting the ongoing association of HIV with death in Japanese popular culture, which assumes that they cannot be "productive" Japanese citizens based on this mischaracterization of HIV/AIDS. Runestad's interviews with a group of men who have struggled in different ways to come to terms with their positive status, and to "live positively," which in the Japanese context translates to meeting a standard model of gendered citizenship based on life course achievements (employment, marriage, family), reveal the ways in which "living positively" simultaneously challenges normative definitions of gendered Japanese citizenship and is impacted by those definitions.

Chapter 7 consists of an ethnographic exploration of a group of long-term (20 or more years) HIV+ gay men aged 60 and older in Toronto who meet fortnightly to discuss and reflect on everyday challenges of living with HIV. Their discussions reveal a critique of the professionalization and biomedical bias in contemporary Canadian HIV/AIDS research and support services, reflecting their shared experiences and memories of profound changes to the HIV/AIDS epidemic in Canada over time. Murray argues that these disengagements with contemporary mainstream Toronto HIV/AIDS organizations (and their attendant discourses about HIV/AIDS), based on shared experiences and memories, produce a particular form of "queer viral time" which challenges taken-for-granted assumptions about the improved "chronic" status of HIV/AIDS, and highlight the importance of biopolitical temporalities in analytical frameworks of the meanings and significance of HIV/AIDS.

Chapter 8 draws from 16 months of ethnographic research on the political and sexual lives of HIV+ poor and working-class Jamaican women. Jolly delineates how organizers of a support group for HIV+ women enact sexual and social intimacies to contest normative moral expectations to "live positively" that require adherence to cultural norms about sexuality, womanhood, and respectability. Jolly observes how this support group develops and cultivates HIV/AIDS care strategies through women-centered networks, such that they can be viewed as intentional communities of interdependence and psychosocial care, rather than being simply invisible "at-risk" groups or passive victims subjected to a paralyzing plague. Jolly also contends that the homosocial intimacies that characterize these networks of care reflect an "intraventive" cultural practice and knowledge, a term that describes the organic ways community members represent and support themselves individually and collectively. This intraventive cultural practice reflects the embodied knowledges of HIV+ Black women and challenges pathologizing public health and academic discourses.

Chapter 9 explores the lives of HIV+ men on ART treatment in urban India: Schensul examines how a group of economically marginal HIV+ men in Mumbai, India, cope with a now chronic, but still serious and highly stigmatized disease, with limited programmatic supports. Through interviews with these men, Schensul examines the impact of an HIV+ status on these men's emotional well-being, spousal relationships, families, finances, and employment. Schensul reveals how these men face multiple stressors in their lives, which are intensified through an HIV diagnosis, and for some of them, lead to higher alcohol intake, which can then lead to problems in ART adherence. Schensul's findings echo and underline Saria's observations about the gap between the "fantasies" of the public health bureaucracy and the individual HIV+ body, and the gap between the state's hegemonic discourses about HIV and everyday life as actually negotiated under immediate constraints of poverty.

The concluding chapter, by Robert Lorway, a leading figure in the anthropology of HIV/AIDS, provides some critical reflections on the preceding chapters. Lorway observes how the contributors to this book force us to think more carefully about the effects of "end of AIDS" and "positive living" narratives by focusing on the new kinds of problems they create for people living with HIV and their carers. Lorway notes the importance of "viral socialities" developed among PLHIV and their supporters during the first decades of the pandemic that produced grassroots activist responses to HIV/AIDS and how these chapters illustrate their gradual disappearance or transformation due in part to the preponderance of HIV elimination narratives premised upon on biomedical interventions, individualized responsibilization discourses, and surveillance data. He urges researchers to explore ongoing and new forms of intimacy and sociality in HIV worlds, which may lead to new forms of PLHIV organization and resistance.

Adia Benton, another leading medical anthropologist specializing in HIV/AIDS, provides some final thoughts on the short- and long-term effects of "End of AIDS" discourses on the governance and management of the pandemic as well as on HIV+ lives. In reflecting on the cumulative impact of the book's chapters, Benton asks us to (re)consider who is "the end of AIDS" (working) for? Who does the discourse serve, and to what uses will it be put? For whom is AIDS to be ending?

NOTES

1. "AIDS-related deaths have been reduced by more than 55% since the peak in 2004. In 2018, around 770 000 [570 000–1.1 million] people died from AIDS-related illnesses worldwide, compared to 1.7 million [1.3 million–2.4 million] in 2004 and 1.2 million [860 000–1.6 million] in 2010." UNAIDS. https://www.unaids.org/en/resources/fact-sheet. Accessed October 16, 2019.

2. https://www.unaids.org/en/topic/treatment accessed October 16, 2019), https://www.unaids.org/en/resources/campaigns/World-AIDS-Day-Report-2014 (accessed October 17, 2019)

3. The development of "Undetectable=Untransmittable" and/or "Treatment as Prevention" campaigns are based on these research findings.

4. At the end of 2019, US$18.6 billion (constant 2016 dollars) was available for the AIDS response in low- and middle-income countries, almost US$1.3 billion less than in 2017 (https://www.unaids.org/en/resources/fact-sheet, accessed September 29, 2020).

5. The authors focusing on this region (Thiongane and Graham) do not reference the specific locations of their research in order to ensure confidentiality and anonymity of participants.

REFERENCES

Benton, Adia, Thurka Sangaramoorthy and Ippolytos Kalofonos. 2017. "Temporality and Positive Living in the Age of HIV/AIDS: A Multisited Ethnography." *Current Anthropology* 58 no. 4: 454–476

Biehl, Joao. 2007. *Will to Live: AIDS Therapies and the Politics of Survival.* Princeton, NJ: Princeton University Press.

Black, Steven P. 2019. *Speech and Song at the Margins of Global Health: Zulu Tradition, HIV Stigma, and AIDS Activism in South Africa.* New Brunswick: Rutgers University Press.

Boellstorff, Tom. 2009. "Nuri's testimony: HIV/AIDS in Indonesia and bare knowledge." *American Ethnologist* 36(2): 351–363.

Boellstorff, Tom. 2011. "But do not identify as gay: A proleptic genealogy of the MSM Category." *Cultural Anthropology* 26(2): 287–312.

Boseley, Sarah and Hannah Devline. 2019. "End to AIDS in sight as huge study finds drugs stop HIV transmission." *The Guardian*, May 2. https://www.theguardian.com/society/2019/may/02/end-to-aids-in-sight-as-huge-study-finds-drugs-stop-hiv-transmission_

Butt, Leslie. 2005. "'Lipstick Girls' and 'Fallen Women': AIDS and conspiratorial thinking in Papua, Indonesia." *Cultural Anthropology* 20(3): 412–442.

Cohen, Jon. 2011. "Halting HIV/AIDS epidemics." *Science* 334(6061): 1338–1340.

Colvin, Christopher J. 2011. "HIV/AIDS, chronic diseases and globalization." *Global Health* 7, no. 31. https://globalizationandhealth.biomedcentral.com/articles/10.1186/1744-8603-7-31.

Colvin, Christopher, Steven Robins and Joan Leavens Joan. 2010. "Grounding 'responsibilisation talk': masculinities, citizenship and HIV in Cape Town, South Africa." *Journal of Development Studies* 46(7): 1179–1195.

Comaroff, Jean. 2007. "Beyond bare life: AIDS, (bio)politics, and the neoliberal order." *Public Culture* 19(1): 197–219.

De Klerk, Josien. 2011. *Being Old in Times of AIDS: Aging, Caring and Relating in Northwest Tanzania.* Leiden, The Netherlands: African Studies Centre.

Farmer, Paul. 2006(1992). *AIDS and Accusation: Haiti and the Geography of Blame.* Berkeley: University of California Press.

Farmer, Paul. 2003. *Pathologies of Power: Health, Human Rights and the New War on the Poor.* Berkeley: University of California Press.

Farmer, Paul. 2001(1999). *Infections and Inequalities: The Modern Plagues.* Berkeley: University of California Press.

Heckert, Carina. 2018. *Fault Lines of Care: Gender, HIV, and Global Health in Bolivia* Rutgers University Press.

Herdt Gilbert. 1987. "AIDS and Anthropology." *Anthropology Today* 3(2): 1–3.

Hirsch, Jennifer, Holly Wardlow, Daniel Jordan Smith, Harriet Phinney, Shanti Parokj, Constance Nathanson, Constance. Eds. 2009. *The Secret: Love, Marriage and HIV.* Nashville: Vanderbilt University Press.

Igonya, Emmy and Eileen Moyer. 2013. "Putting sex on the table: sex, sexuality, and masculinity among HIV positive men in Nairobi, Kenya." *Culture, Health and Sexuality.* 15(Suppl. 4): S567–S580.

Jolivette, Andrew J. 2016. *Indian Blood: HIV and Trauma in San Francisco's Two-Spirit Community.* Seattle: University of Washington Press.

Kenworthy, Nora. 2017. *Mistreated: The Political Consequences of the Fight Against AIDS in Lesotho.* Nashville: Vanderbilt University Press.

Kerrigan, Deanna and Clare Barrington (Eds.) 2018. *Structural Dynamics of HIV: Risk, Resilience and Response.* Cham, Switzerland: Springer.

Lorway, Robert. 2017. *AIDS Activism, Science and Community Across Three Continents.* Basel: Springer International Publishing.

MacQueen Kathleen M. 1994. "The epidemiology of HIV transmission: trends, structure and dynamics." *Annual Review of Anthropology* 23: 509–526.

Manderson, Lenore and Caroline Smith-Morris. 2010. *Chronic conditions, fluid states: Chronicity and the Anthropology of Illness.* New Brunswick, NJ: Rutgers University Press.

Marten, Meredith. 2020. "Living with HIV as Donor Aid Declines in Tanzania." *Medical Anthropology* 39 (3): 197–210.

McGrath, Janet W., Margaret S. Winchester, David Kaawa-Mafigiri, Eddy Walakira, Florence Namutiibwa, Judith Birungi, George Ssendegye, Amina Nalwoga, Emily Kyarikunda, Sheila Kisakye, Nicolas Ayebazibwe and Charles B. Rwabukwali. 2014. "Challenging the paradigm: anthropological perspectives on HIV as a chronic disease." *Medical Anthropology* 33(4): 303–317.

McKinley, Jesse. "New York Says End of AIDS Epidemic Is Near." *The New York Times*, October 2. Accessed October 15, 2019. https://www.nytimes.com/2019/10/02/nyregion/aids-hiv-epidemic-ny.html

Moyer, Ellen. 2012. "Faidha Gani? What's the point: HIV and the logics of (non)-disclosure among young activists in Zanzibar." *Culture, Health and Sexuality* 14(Suppl. 1): 67–79.

Moyer, Ellen. 2015. "The anthropology of life after AIDS: Epistemological continuities in the age of antiretroviral treatment." *Annual Review of Anthropology* 44: 259–275.

Murray, David. A.B. 2020. "Pozitively Me: HIV support groups, culture and individualism in Toronto." *Medical Anthropology*, DOI: 10.1080/01459740.2020.1711754

Mykhalovskiy, Eric and M. Rosengarten. 2009. "HIV/AIDS in its third decade: Renewed Critique in social and cultural analysis: an introduction." *Social Theory & Health* 7: 187–195.

Mykhalovskiy, Eric, and Viviane Namaste (Eds.), 2019. *Thinking Differently About HIV/AIDS: Contributions from Critical Social Science* (Vancouver, UBC Press)

Nguyen, Vinh Kim. 2005. "Uses and Pleasures: Sexual Modernity, HIV/AIDS, and Confessional Technologies in a West African Metropolis." In *Sex in Development: Science, Sexuality, and Morality in Global Perspective*. Stacey Pigg, ed. 245–68.

Nguyen Vinh-Kim. 2010. *The Republic of Therapy: Triage and Sovereignty in West Africa's Time of AIDS*. Durham, NC: Duke University Press.

Nguyen Vinh-Kim, N. Bajos, F. Dubois-Arber, J. O'Malley and CM Pirkle. 2011. "Remedicalizing an epidemic: from HIV treatment as prevention to HIV treatment as prevention." *AIDS* 25(3): 291–293.

O'Daniel, Alyson. 2016. *Holding On: African American Women Surviving HIV/AIDS*. Lincoln: University of Nebraska Press.

Patton, Cindy. 1990. *Inventing AIDS*. New York: Routledge.

Patton ,Cindy. 2002. *Globalizing AIDS*. Minneapolis: University of Minnesota Press.

Pigg, Stacy Leigh. 2001. "Languages of Sex and AIDS in Nepal: Notes on the Social Production of Commensurability." *Cultural Anthropology*, 16: 481–541.

Public Health Agency of Canada. 2017 *Statement on behalf of the Council of Chief Medical Officers of Health*, November 30, 2017. https://www.canada.ca/en/publichealth/news/2017/11/statement_on_behalfofthecouncilofchiefmedicalofficersofhealth.html

Reed, Joel Christian. 2018. *Landscapes of Activism: Civil Society, HIV and AIDS Care in Northern Mozambique*. New Brunswick: Rutgers University Press, 2018.

Rourke, Sean and Bill Flanagan. 2020. "The end of the HIV crisis is within our grasp. We must apply the pandemic spirit to achieve it." *The Globe and Mail*. August 27, 2020. https://www.theglobeandmail.com/opinion/article-the-end-of-the-hiv-crisis-is-within-our-grasp-we-must-apply-the/#comments

Sangaramoorthy, Thurka. 2014. *Treating AIDS: Politics of Difference, Paradox of Prevention* New Brunswick, NJ: Rutgers University Press.

Sangaramoorthy, Thurka. 2018. "Chronicity, Crisis and the 'End of AIDS.'" *Global Public Health* 13(1): 1–15.

Seeley, Janet. 2014. *HIV and East Africa: Thirty Years in the Shadow of an Epidemic*. London: Routledge.

Singer, Merrill, C. Flores, L. Davidson, G. Burke, Z. Castillo et al. 1990. "The economic, social and cultural context of AIDS among Latinos." *Medical Anthropology Quarterly* 4(1): 72–114.

Smith, Daniel Jordan. 2014. *AIDS Doesn't Show Its Face: Inequality, Morality, and Social Change in Nigeria*. Chicago: University of Chicago Press.

Smith, Daniel and Benjamin Mbakwem. 2010. "Antiretroviral therapy and reproductive life projects: mitigating the stigma of AIDS in Nigeria." *Social Science and Medicine*. 71(2): 345–352.

Sobo, Elise J. 1999. "Editorial: Cultural models and HIV/AIDS: new anthropological views." *Anthropology and Medicine* 6(1): 5–12.

Treichler, Paula. 1999. *How to Have Theory in an Epidemic: Cultural Chronicles of AIDS*. Durham: Duke University Press.

Vernooij, E., M. Mehlo, A. Hardon and R. Reis. 2016. "Access for all: Contextualising HIV treatment as prevention in Swaziland." *AIDS Care* 28 (supp.3): 7–13.

Wardlow, Holly. 2008. "'She liked it best when she was on top': Intimacies and Estrangements in Huli Men's Marital and Extramarital Relationships." In William Jankowiak (ed.), *Intimacies: Love and Sex across Cultures*, pp. 194–223. New York: Columbia University Press.

Watkins-Hayes, Celeste. 2014. "Intersectionality and the Sociology of HIV/AIDS: Past, Present, and Future Research Directions." *Annual Review of Sociology* 40: 431–457.

Whyte, Suzanne Reynolds, ed. 2014. *Second Chances: Surviving AIDS in Uganda*. Durham: Duke University Press.

Yingling, Thomas. 1997. *AIDS and the National Body*. Durham, NC: Duke University Press.

Part I

FANTASTIC CONCEITS AND HOW TO MIND THEM

MANAGING PLHIV IN "POST-CRISIS" TIMES

Chapter 1

Forty Years of AIDS

Fatigue, Failure, and Fantasies

Vaibhav Saria

In December 2018, some of the major English dailies in India reported that a 24-year-old pregnant woman in Madurai had contracted HIV through a blood transfusion. The young woman was pregnant with her second child and had been advised to get a blood transfusion because of a hemoglobin deficiency (Press Trust of India 2018a). This type of scandal, as well as ones relating to drug shortages at antiretroviral therapy (ART) centers and discrimination against HIV+ children who are denied admission to schools, pops up frequently in Indian news and then disappear as quickly, evidencing the leaky, overwhelmed public health infrastructure as much as the continuing sensationalism associated with the disease. What made the incident in Madurai linger on in the media for days was the fact the young donor, a 19-year-old factory worker, attempted to kill himself by consuming rat poison after he learned he was HIV+ and heard the news of the pregnant woman's infection (Press Trust of India, 2018b); he was rushed to the hospital where he died three days later (Outlook Web Bureau 2018). When further inquiries were made, it was discovered not only that the blood had not been screened properly but also that the young man had actually tested positive for HIV as far back as 2016 when he had donated blood on a previous occasion (Sundar 2018). Although a counselor had tried to reach him, he was out of town and the case was not followed up. Some news reports also mentioned that he had tested positive for HIV on yet another occasion during which he had had routine blood work done to secure a visa to go abroad for a job.

This quick succession of events reveals the impossibility of reducing HIV (or any pathogen for that matter) to a biological phenomenon: one positive diagnosis of HIV gets linked to a contaminated blood supply chain, an overworked and underpaid counselor working in a cash-strapped public health system, a suicide, histories of migration from South Asia for employment, international laws barring HIV+ people from immigrating, and finally, to bureaucratically presupposed conceptions of a good life. This dramatic and tragic narrative of the disclosure of a diagnosis that is not only medical but freighted with legal, political, and criminal implications is also a good way to begin an assessment of the epidemic in India. This chapter will look at how the epidemic is tackled in multiple sites, such as the Indian state's ART supply chain and the private provider's clinic, and by multiple actors including people belonging to the so-called high-risk population.[1] This broad canvas shows how—in the context of poverty in India—HIV continues to be determined by the same kinds of failure and mismanagement as previous and ongoing pandemics such as tuberculosis and famines. This produced crisis predictably intensifies fear of death and dying (social and otherwise), which in turn influences how health care providers manage people living with HIV (PLHIV). The manufactured crisis also promotes a sense of fatigue that is reflected in how "high-risk" populations face the intractable challenges of living with HIV. The findings presented were collected across multiple projects and sites in India between 2008 and 2019 where I conducted interviews and participant observation in doctors' clinics, shadowed HIV counselors, and interviewed PLHIV.

ART IN INDIA

One of the foundational stories of the global fight against HIV is how generic ART came to save the day. The production of affordable medicines was made possible through the exceptions established in international patent laws, a rare occurrence in which the logic of the market was forced to align with the ethical horizons of global health. Yet a look at how the Indian public sector manages the treatment of the 2.1 million PLHIV reveals fraught and fragile treatment opportunities. The HIV epidemic in India is overseen by the National AIDS Control Organization (NACO), which in turn oversees the 35 state-run AIDS control societies (SACs), which oversee the 189 District AIDS Prevention Control Units (DAPCUs) that were established in high-priority areas. These DAPCUs also have at their disposal 105 mobile Integrated Counseling and Testing Units (ICTU) that enable them to reach hotspots that are up to 30 kilometers away from the brick and mortar DAPCUs. This organizational structure is responsible for, among other things, ensuring that medicines reach people who are living with HIV. Yet the production of generic medicines within India's own borders has not ensured the availability of ART primarily because of competing logics: while public welfare demands fixed lower prices, the private market demands profit for the pharmaceutical industry to thrive (Lalitha 2014, Milard et al. 2018, Srinivasan et al. 2013).

The availability of funds through global health initiatives has provided an excuse for the Government of India to constantly slash monies allocated for drug procurement, forcing the Global Fund to step in to fill the gap (Mahajan 2008).[2]

Despite having access to generic medications and ART's affordability, until 2018 the Indian government used domestic funds to procure less than 50% of ART (PEPFAR India 2017, 38; World Bank 2013). Most of the funding for ART in India came from the Global Fund and through the World Bank. At the national fiscal level at least, HIV was a source of valuable foreign income rather than domestic expenditure.[3] Whether a person with HIV gets ART in their hands, however, is not solely determined by the government's desire for financial profit, but the availability of foreign funds has allowed for the government to not invest domestic funds for the epidemic. This meant that the Indian state was not pressured into creating or strengthening the supply chain system of ART in the public sector that has long been the bane of PLHIV in India. Generic ART is acquired by NACO and then distributed to the SACs, the DAPCUs, and the mobile ICTUs through a tender-and-bidding system. The DAPCUs submit estimates of proposed ART needs; these estimates are then aggregated and tenders released by the Ministry of Health and Family Welfare, after which bids are received by private companies. The company that wins the bids then supplies the medicine. The process that was in place for procuring medications until 2013 is outlined in figure 1.1.[4]

This model for procuring drugs, not surprisingly, led to many bottlenecks and to ongoing complaints of drug shortages in many of the ART centers across the country, creating additional challenges for PLHIV. Not only is the much-lauded generic ART not made available to patients immediately owing to the competitive pricing, tender, and bidding process the government engages in, but given that brand-name drugs are often rebranded as generic government medicines to make them available as public sector products, this supply chain has more to do with the state wanting to appear to be in beneficent control, rather than improving actual affordability or efficacy. This supply chain setup is not particular to the management of HIV but is borrowed from the management of the much older and persistent tuberculosis epidemic (Nichter 2020), malaria, and existing vaccination programs (Department of Health and Family Welfare 2016, 10).

Attempts to decentralize the supply chain system led to the establishment of Central Medical Services Society (CMSS) in 2012 as the central procurement agency of the Ministry of Health and Family Welfare, the aim of which was to ensure that the procurement of all health sector goods was separated from other bureaucratic responsibilities and was delegated to one state company. The launch of CMSS was accompanied with much hope and hype about new technologies that promised rapid information sharing—of projected demands,

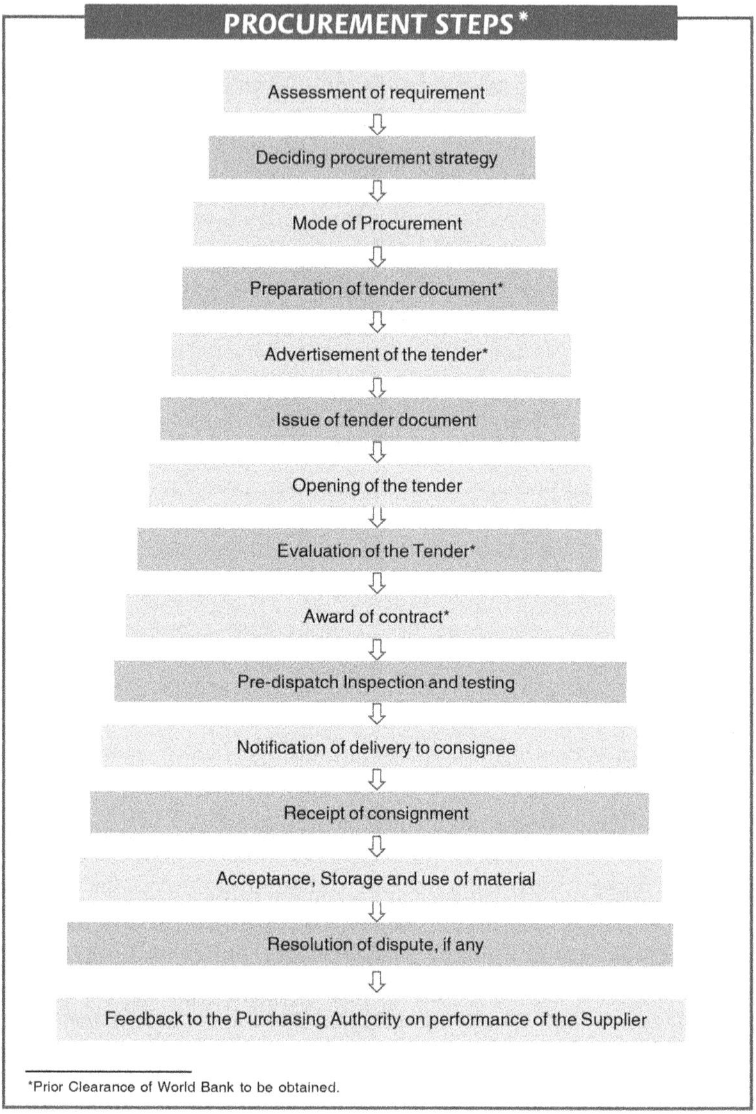

Figure 1.1 NACO Procurement Steps for ART under Phase 3 of the National AIDS Control Program. *Source*: *Procurement Manual for NACP-III* (2007, 14). Government of India.

past use, and other issues concerning spoilage and storage—through an IT-enabled infrastructure that would harness the power of advanced computing via the Center for Development of Advanced Computing (a department under the Ministry of Electronics and Information Technology). One reason the CMSS was created was to address the shrinking resources from global health organizations, as these organizations, along with the Bill and Melinda Gates Foundation and the Clinical Health Access Initiative, began phasing out supplying resources to fight HIV/AIDS in 2015 (PEPFAR 2017, 10). Improving the supply chain was a condition set forth by the World Bank for extending its financial support, and it is considered crucial for the Indian government's transition to complete management of the epidemic by 2020.[5]

However, the decentralization of CMSS has not solved the problem of drug shortages for the millions of patients being treated in the public sector, thus compelling patients to shift to the equally vast but patchily regulated private sector (Bhat 1996). That these shortages are reported frequently in the Indian media in a matter-of-fact way indicates that they are not a surprising exception but par for the course. For example, in 2014, it was reported:

> A delayed tendering process for antiretroviral drugs by the Indian National AIDS Control Organisation (NACO) meant that 150,000 people living with HIV (PLHIV) in India were at risk of being without antiretroviral treatment (ART) for October. . . . Some Indian pharmaceutical companies have called an emergency situation, halting the production of other drugs to meet the immediate demand for the antiretroviral drugs. . . . The drug shortage in this instance was the result of a delayed tendering process in the government's procurement of the drugs meant that sign-off of the drug combination tenofovir/lamivudine hadn't happened until mid September. (Reuters 2014)

Drug shortages and stockouts in India owing to changes in drug combinations or formulas have characterized the Indian experience of HIV/AIDS ever since generic ART first became available (Bhuyan 2018; Jain and Stephens 2008).

The drug shortages that result from the byzantine ART supply chain system in India not only make everyday life more difficult for the majority of PLHIV, an overwhelming number of whom are poor and who rely on the Indian public health delivery system, but also have a bearing on why the young man in Madurai committed suicide almost 40 years after the first HIV case was detected. The HIV epidemic remains an emergency, but more importantly, it has long been and continues to be a manufactured emergency due to the unrealistic ways it gets incorporated into the agendas of the nation-state, fiscal and otherwise. The manufactured aspect of this crisis in India also has precedence in other historical and ongoing crises such as famines that were solely the consequence of the state's public distribution systems (Dreze and Sen 1990). It is valuable to analyze the HIV epidemic against the background context of other health crises in the subcontinent because the history of the management of such crises has direct bearing on how health care providers manage their HIV+ patients.

DRUG-RESISTANT CULTURES

While shadowing health care providers in the city of Patna in the eastern state of Bihar in India between 2014 and 2018, I witnessed the following clinical encounter between Dr. T, who was well known in the city as an HIV specialist, and his patient. The wall of his examination room in the ground floor of a building was covered floor to ceiling with professional certificates he had collected over 20 years of attending various HIV training sessions and HIV continuing medical education seminars organized by pharmaceutical companies, NGOs, and the Bihar State AIDS Control Society. The patient was a middle-aged man who had been in the care of Dr. T but then moved to Bombay for a job for a period of many months, during which time he had not been receiving the first-line ART that Dr. T had prescribed. Upon his return to Patna, having become too ill to continue working, Dr. T prescribed the patient a second-line antiretroviral therapy (ART) treatment, and he was at Dr. T's that day for a checkup.

Dr. T: You have come after such a long gap. You've come back after one and a half years, even though you know your regimen is a complicated one. You were part of the first-line ART program, but after such a gap, you now have been pushed to the second line. You should not miss appointments either when you are on medication, because when you are on treatment we have to see if your medicines are getting metabolized, what the effects they are having on your liver, what effects they are having are on your cholesterol, what effects they are having on your kidneys. It is very important to know these things, and you had trouble walking, didn't you? Have you been taking these medications or have you stopped altogether?

Patient: I was taking them before the prescription ran out.

Dr. T: And you were taking two medicines, one of them every morning and every evening, plus the other one once a day?

Patient: No, I was just taking one pill.

Dr. T: Which one?

Patient: Let me show you.

Dr. T: Where did you vanish to for so long?

Patient: I went to Bombay.

Dr. T: Did you go for work?

Patient: Yes, I was there for about ten months.

Dr. T: You should have gone to the ART center in Bombay at least.

Patient: Since I returned, I have been taking Zidolam.

Dr. T: Twice a day, right?

Patient: Yes.

Dr. T: And this Virataz, are you still taking this?

Patient: No, you had asked me to stop taking that.

Dr. T: No! I had marked this red, which doesn't mean you stop taking it but that you should never stop taking it. You are supposed to take Zidolam twice, morning and evening, and Virataz once a day. You've just been taking half your medicines on the second line. After this, there will be very few options left for you, and you will be in grave trouble.

Patient: I had become completely well.

Dr. T: This is the mistake you made. I had taken so much time to explain to you that you cannot neglect these medicines. You tell me honestly, whether I had explained everything to you or not?

Writing down a new treatment regimen for the patient, Dr. T asked: "Did you think that because you're feeling okay, you should stop the medications?" The patient replied that the medicines were very expensive and he could not afford to buy them in Bombay. Dr. T then replied exasperatedly, "If you had told me, I would have had your paperwork transferred to the Bombay ART center." When the patient left, Dr. T turned to me and said: "Look, he stopped taking the medicines by himself, and I don't believe that he had problems with money. His income source is the same now as it was then. He doesn't have the burden of arranging marriages for sons and daughters. He just took my advice very lightly. This is the problem, they feel fine, so they stop taking the medications."

This clinical encounter not only highlights the gap between the official discourse of HIV and its lived reality but also illustrates how the concept of HIV is given life in different contexts. The patient complained of a system that had failed him by making it difficult to seamlessly transfer HIV treatment across states and cities. This is a glaring—even if unsurprising—problem given the large number of migrant populations in India, populations that have been the focus of HIV prevention and treatment programs. Yet Dr. T insisted that the patient did not understand the notion of sticking with a treatment regimen. When I pressed Dr. T on why patients do not understand compliance with regimens, especially given how rising cases of diabetes and hypertension in India across class lines over the last 40 years have made compliance a familiar notion, Dr. T mumbled something about stigma. The patient signaled that it was impossible to maintain an ART regimen because of the complicated bureaucracy of local health systems, whereas Dr. T mystified noncompliance through excuses such as illiteracy and a fear of stigma that have become idiomatic in describing the poor in India. Veena Das and Ranendra Das (2007) have cautioned against too quickly pointing to patients as the problem when they do not adhere to or complete treatments when it is often the bureaucratic workings of the public sector, with its emphasis on standardized protocols, that fail patients. As Foucault (1980) reminds us, public health immediately became a matter of policing and financing when it emerged as a discipline in the eighteenth century. The Indian state's response to the epidemic has been characterized by surveillance, decentralization, profiteering, *and* funding difficulties, which have affected supply chains and patient compliance.[6] Yet the failure to live healthily with HIV is placed squarely on patients' shoulders.

THE DAMAGES OF A DIAGNOSIS

To better understand why the young blood donor committed suicide after being diagnosed with HIV in 2018, we can turn to yet another clinical encounter. Dr. A, who served the poor inhabiting the urban peripheries of Patna, told me the following account in the first interview I conducted with him (then repeated several times subsequently as I shadowed him in his clinic). A young man who used to work as an unlicensed assistant for another doctor—a friend of Dr. A—had been dismissed from his job because he had been diagnosed as positive for HIV. He had come to ask Dr. A for a job. When Dr. A inquired why he was seeking a new job, the young man explained what had happened and showed him the test result. Dr. A told him that he did not think the young man had HIV, that the test looked unreliable to him. Dr. A then asked the young man to get another test; he then called the lab beforehand and instructed it to disregard the actual results and tell the young man that his results were negative. The man went back to see Dr. A, who said to him: "See, you don't have HIV. Go to your village, exercise every morning, eat well." Three months later, when the man returned to visit Dr. A, he had gained 10 kilos. Dr. A explained his intentions to me: "When a man's mind is strong he can withstand anything. When he is scared, he dies from the worry before the illness. Our mind is like a Pandora's box; what may come out of it once opened? As it is, we are all going to die, why must you die by being suffocated by fear? Why die every day?" Dr. A's outlook on how to help his patients live with HIV is both troubling and powerful. Troubling for obvious reasons, in view of its untruthfulness, yet powerful because of the way it reveals the massive damage wrought by fear when living with HIV in the context of poverty.

In his analysis of the bareback porn film *Viral Loads*, Tim Dean describes a controversial scene that may help us better understand the clinical encounters in Patna. The scene shows a jar of 200 loads of semen from HIV+ men squirted up the pornstar's ass. "In the film," Dean explains, "the jar of liquid is clearly marked on its lid with the words 'poz cum.' . . . Now, of course, HIV is killed by exposure to air; semen stored in a jar would not be infectious. The scene is not enacting a risk but hyperbolically staging a fantasy" (2015, 241). The metaphor of staging is revealing not only for understanding this porn scene but it also provides a parallel means of understanding the

Indian government's approach to the HIV crisis, as the state "stages" a story about HIV that in fact enacts risk for the poor. The state's way of managing the epidemic—staging HIV in the Indian context as a challenge defined by scarcity, precarity, and a severe threat to living—helps to explain the suicide of the young man described at the beginning of the chapter. It might prove useful to remember that the young man who committed suicide was trying to migrate abroad for work, an important way to earn a livelihood and sustain families back home through remittances. Dr. T.'s patient was also a migrant laborer who worked in Bombay but returned home when he was no longer able to work because of his illness, and Dr. A's patient likewise lost his job because of his diagnosis.

These cases alert us to how the state's performance in the area of HIV treatment and support does not reflect the everyday lived realities of the urban or migrating poor; it is instead governed by ambitions of cost-effectiveness and social control. There is a fatal disconnect between the imaginary of the bureaucratic state and the actuality on the ground. A disconnect that both stems from and feeds into the distinct fantasies under which the different actors of the HIV network function. Indeed, the extent to which fantasy has underwritten the approach to the HIV epidemic is one of the durable lessons of queer theory's critical study of it. Leo Bersani, in his now iconic essay "Is the Rectum a Grave?" (1987), studies the infamous Ray brothers incident, asking why a group of residents in Arcadia, Florida, "set fire to the house of the Ray family with three hemophiliac children" who had been infected with HIV (199). His answer was that the Arcadia residents did not see the Ray brothers as they were, namely, as three HIV+ straight hemophiliac boys; instead, to the citizens they "unconsciously represented the infinitely more seductive and intolerable image of a grown man, legs high in the air, unable to refuse the suicidal ecstasy of being a woman" (212). Bersani's description of the sexual meaning of HIV infection assumed by the public helps us understand Dr. A's explanation as to why he sought to undo the damages of a HIV+ diagnosis by undoing the diagnosis itself. For the patients whose stories I have presented here, and for the young blood donor who killed himself, HIV consciously and unconsciously represents not only a matter of sexuality but of insurmountable difficulties that make living impossible.

Dr. A assumed that HIV for the urban poor results in being "suffocated by fear" and it entails "dying every day," and because "our mind is like a Pandora's box" it is impossible to control or tolerate these fears and fantasies that have a high possibility of becoming actualized because of the material conditions created by the state. Another iconic essay, by Cathy J. Cohen, "Punks, Bulldaggers, and Welfare Queens: The Radical Potential of Queer Politics?" (1997), shifted the binary between normal and pathologized sexuality from hetero-versus-homo to the kind of sexualities the state encourages versus the ones that the state penalizes. Using this lens allows us to understand the relationship that racialized and poor bodies have with the state as pathologized, and brings us closer to understanding what HIV represents for the state, the state's actors, and the infected urban poor in India. Dr. A's idea of the everyday world of PLHIV as a site that needs to be sustained and protected—from the fantasies of the state and psychic fears among patients alike—has important implications for how HIV is conceived in the clinics of India.

Philosopher Jocelyn Benoist offers an example of how concepts gain life in the context in which they are used, explaining that while an apple sorbet might not look like an apple, something like an apple flavor can be recognized in it, thus constituting a "living concept" of an apple (2010). The way HIV comes alive or becomes a living concept in the clinic is not only through hard scientific facts but also through the fears and worries over conditions of living that it gives rise to. The conception of HIV in the clinic reveals how clinic staff was imagining in patients a form of life rather than seeing them solely as bearers of disease—a form of life that was born into a world with the odds already stacked against them, for example, a broken public distribution system that was responsible for famine, hunger, and starvation long before it also started making it difficult to access ART. Applying the implications of Benoist's notion of a living concept for everyday life to the urban poor, Veena Das argues that by looking at how concepts come to life differently in different contexts, we see "possibility as an essential feature of the real." Das writes, "Harmony between thought and reality" does not lie "in correctly specifying the referent of a concept but rather in understanding that possibility may well provide the footing within which actuality can be reality" (2020, 156). Dr. A and to a certain extent Dr. T were both well aware what HIV signified in scientific language and how it was staged in the public health system of India; hence, they were also aware of the difficulties that a diagnosis causes for poor migrant laborers in Bihar. Both of them were in some ways attempting to effect a harmony between the imaginary and the reality of HIV by directing their patients to another possibility of living with HIV. Once Dr. A's patient was relieved of the suffocating fear of HIV, he stopped dying every day and a different reality was actualized. While the concepts of staging and everyday life stem from Erving Goffman's study *The Presentation of Self in Everyday Life* (1978), the everyday, Das reminds us, is the space where devastation takes place and also the place that one has to inhabit again "by putting together the rubble and ruins," a crafting made possible through ordinary ethical action (61). Ordinary ethics like the kind Dr. A applied in the case of his patient reveals that "reality here is deeply contextual—one has neither a frontal view of reality as if it were before our eyes nor a relativist view as if death could be conceptualized and grasped rather than being the searing singular event" (155). The deeply contextual reality that Dr. A showed he understood is reformulated in other ways as well vis-à-vis HIV in India, as we shall see now in the case of Dr. B. M. Hegde.

Dr. Hegde was cited by many doctors during my fieldwork as a source of inspiration in helping them think about how they deal with patients who are confronting potentially devastating diagnoses such as HIV. Hegde is a much celebrated and decorated physician who won the Padma Bhushan, the Indian state's third highest civilian honor, in 2010. He has long controversially argued that AIDS in India should be relabeled NIDS (Nutritional Immune Deficiency Syndrome) (2011, 2012). Many aspects of Dr. Hegde's argument have drawn the ire of fellow scientists and doctors who dismiss him as a quack because his claims are not based on any research. While Dr. Hegde is not denying that HIV is a viral infection, his setting up of a confrontation between malnutrition and HIV is clearly unnecessary. Dr. Hegde's influence among other doctors can be explained by the fact that he was trained in Western biomedicine and at respectable institutions inside and outside India. This training has allowed him to present another facet of reality that resonates more with the doctors in the clinics where I worked. "Poverty, with its consequent nutritional deficiency, does not seem to be easing in the near future," he noted around 2010, and continued to write that "Economist Utsa Patnaik in her lecture recently in Chennai testified that between 1991 and 2001, the first post-liberalisation decade, the per capita consumption of food grains had gone down by at least 25 to 30 kgs. 75% of protein and calorie energy come from food grains for the rural poor; the fall in consumption will have serious impact on their nutritional status." This, he added, would "impact the childhood malnutrition load seriously" (n.d., 77). Hegde's efforts to show how something as fundamental and widespread as nutrition underwrites the AIDS crisis anchors HIV to variables other than sexuality. In some ways, Hegde is echoing critiques that have been made against single-disease interventions, the predominant design of AIDS prevention and treatment championed by global health (Birn 2014; Engelmann and Kehr 2014; Mahajan 2018). Hegde and other doctors in Patna underscore the gap between the realities faced by the clinic's patients and the global discourse surrounding HIV. By emphasizing the everyday and a temporality associated with nutrition rather than HIV, Dr. A, the patients in Dr. T's clinic, and Hegde all point to a critical gap between hegemonic HIV discourses and the lives of urban poor migrants in Bihar, reminding us that "discourse is not life, its time is not your time" (Foucault 1991, 72).

Although the alternative realities being crafted by Dr. A in his clinic, and by Dr. Hegde more publicly, resulted from their ethical engagement with HIV, they remain troubling and inadequate because they sustain assumptions about the poor that have remained a constant since the start of the HIV epidemic, at least in India. Poor patients are framed as ignorant, unable to understand the importance of the ART daily regimen, and as bearing a fear of being HIV+ that remains beyond counseling—these and related assumptions reproduce the state's fantasy of the poor that are routinely articulated to explain failure to live with HIV.[7] Nowhere is this fantasy more clearly seen than in Dr. Hegde's claims which, very much like the claim that poor patients are not capable of handling the fear of HIV, demonstrates how the state is incapable of confronting the realities of HIV.

SEXUALITY AND POVERTY

Though Hegde does not mention sexuality in his polemics, his work can be read as a version of Adam Geary's masterful treatment of scientific material showing how anxieties regarding sexuality render invisible the racialized aspects of the HIV epidemic in the United States. Geary points to histories of nutritional deficiency, incarceration, and geographies of poverty to explain the high rates of HIV infection among African Americans and to argue for a molecular understanding of HIV rather than a sexual one (2014). In rural India, HIV as negotiated was interpreted by some as evidence of deviant sexuality, but not by others. For example, a young man walked into Dr. T.'s clinic and began, "Sir, I had *galat sambhog* [wrongful sexual interaction]," and Dr. T stopped him immediately with a wave of his hand and started asking him about his symptoms, prescribed an HIV test and some antibiotics, and asked him to come again with the results. Yet another scared patient tried to say, "I promise I won't do it again," but Dr. T was not interested and just turned to me in conversation. Dr. A saw an ailing young man accompanied by his scared wife; the wife whispered to Dr. A that her husband got HIV in Bombay, but Dr. A was not interested and just said, "Yes, okay," and proceeded to prescribe medicines and a test. I could have wrongly been led to believe that sexuality was excusable for providers, but my earlier research on hijras (one of India's "third gendered" population) made me aware that providers understood the sexuality of men as natural and excusable as contrasted with the sexuality of trans women (Saria 2015a, 2015b).

To look at for whom and how HIV was received as a sexual disease, I turn to my fieldwork among hijras that I conducted between 2008 and 2018 in rural Orissa, a state in Eastern India. *Hijra* is a term now translated as "transgenders" in Indian English, and in the epidemiological literature hijras are described as men who have sex with men (MSM). They are discursively framed as a population at high risk for HIV, but they have not been the beneficiary of the kindness that doctors in Patna show to their clients who are men, and they elicit curiosity in the DAPCUs whenever they go to get their test results. A counselor in Bhadrak asked me, "Are they really incapable of loving women?" I said, "Yes, a lot of people across the world feel the same way they do." The counselor replied, "So they don't even love their mothers?" to which I responded, "No, they love their mothers, but they don't love their mothers sexually." Hijras in Bhadrak and Kalahandi (in rural Eastern India) had been recruited as local experts to spread the gospel of safer sex and positive living, yet they themselves came to realize that they could not aspire to those goals. One evening, as Pawan Hijra was sadly recounting her visit to the deathbed of a fellow hijra, Jasmine (also a hijra) started dancing energetically. She then turned to us and said: "All of this is just in the mind. You think positively, you live healthily—look at me dancing, I have so much energy—you live happily and with energy your CD4 won't drop." Pawan Hijra and I smiled at her ruefully. Jasmine was trying to do for herself what Dr. A did for his young patient. Jasmine refused to frame her sexuality as a site of intervention and saw it as integral and unyielding—just as doctors did for their male patients. Jasmine once told me, "I am not sure what it is, but no matter what, the itch to get fucked never goes away. Sometimes I shove my own fingers in, and you are talking about insisting on condoms. In the middle of the night, who will wait if you don't have a condom, if you have the itch?" Jasmine was illustrating how sexuality was presented as amenable to change and control in HIV prevention discourse, when it wasn't experienced that way by many. The resistance to such a discourse, which set up hijras to fail as good HIV subjects, is seen by her emphasizing the importance of a "good mindset." Thus, even in the context of poverty, excuses and explanations for sexuality were differentially distributed and weighted depending on the gendered body.

In other words, while the state's management of HIV at one level affected everybody who was living with HIV equally, in the field the epidemic came to be received very differently despite the shared local moral world of poverty in rural India. For hijras, despite our knowledge of the faulty supply chain system and the history of nutritional deficiencies, HIV still functioned under the sign of sexuality and consequently hijras understanding of it tied our sexuality to a very specific revelatory analytic of blood and routes of infection. Desires emerged from the perception of a body that could not accommodate sexuality and prevent infection at the same time. Foreskins and anuses that would tear without any available lubricant, and the subsequent appearance of blood that would make us wonder whether that had been the fatal fuck. The specificity of this perception emerged from the fact that HIV in our blood would be read as evidence of our sexuality. Although the anxiety of HIV was not only present for hijras but also for other villagers, for the latter the analytic of blood did not implicate a transgressive gender and sexuality and hence HIV transmission was imagined very differently.

Men in Bhadrak would frequently stop the DAPCU office manager on the street to ask whether one could contract HIV from getting a shave at the barbershops that dotted the district highway. "No," he would say, "HIV dies as soon as exposed to air; don't worry, it does not live even five seconds," then he would count "one, two, three, four, five," but despite his explaining it many times, the idea that it was possible to contract HIV that way persisted. In one of the very first ethnographic interviews I conducted in 2008, in a hospital in Calcutta, the brother of the HIV+ patient insisted that he got it by going to the barbers: "You know they might not have changed the blade. My brother is a very good man, has not done anything wrong." At that time I casually dismissed this as way of shielding the family and the patient from the shame and stigma that that would arise with questions about his sexuality. Nearly a decade later I reinterpreted these explanations as revealing a different imagination of risk, blood, and HIV transmission. I was analyzing interviews that had been conducted as part of the DREAMS (Determined, Resilient, Empowered, AIDS-Free, Mentored, and Safe) initiative that sought to conduct implementation research to measure the feasibility of introducing preexposure prophylaxis (PrEP) to adolescent girls and young women in 10 sub-Saharan countries (Pilgrim et al. 2018). In one of the interviews, a father in Tanzania who was asked whether he would allow his young daughter to take PrEP replied: "Of course, HIV does not just happen through sex. If there is a car accident and my daughter goes to help the victims, she herself might get infected through cuts; she would not know whether the person she is helping has HIV." The interviewer refused to engage with this analytic of blood and directed the conversation back to sexuality by asking whether the father would have any concerns about promiscuity or sex before marriage.

Whether or not HIV can be transmitted through shaving blades or car accidents is beside the point, but this analytic of blood reveals how health and risk are imagined as attached to ordinary activities for the poor. Yet global health systems employ clinical language comprising keywords, categories, and classificatory schemes referring to key populations, high-risk behavior, which keeps HIV intact as evidence of deviant sexuality in blood. Chevrier and their colleagues (2016) illustrate this moral impulse on the part of global health to police sexuality in their description of a STD clinic in Karnataka. The authors first describe the attempts of an organization led by sex workers to establish a community care center, a proposal that was knocked down because the sex worker organization was not seen as an appropriate partner for the delivery of HIV treatment services. However, this distinction between general and key populations is a fiction of scientific discourse: when the organization finally did establish a STD clinic on its own, its staff was surprised to welcome PLHIV who were not sex workers or members of key populations. When Chevrier and their coauthors inquired why this general population with HIV came to a sex worker clinic, their informants told them it was because the sex workers' STD clinic offered nondiscriminatory services. HIV has been a stage on which the state, the clinic, and the law play out their fantasies of policing deviant sexuality, and as this fantasy bears little relation to reality on the ground it is not surprising that the construction of "general versus key populations" with respect to HIV does not hold. According to global health systems, there is no general population living with HIV because HIV will always be attached to deviant sexuality and not to hemophilia, barbers' shaving blades, or car accidents. Thus, global health maintains HIV/AIDS as an epidemic concentrated among "key populations" by absorbing members of the general population into it through its structure of metrics and risk reporting.[8] Ironically, because of the differential manner in which sexuality was excused in the clinic, the discourse of HIV/AIDS ends up making sexual minorities more vulnerable by interpellating their gender and sexuality as risky.

Robert Lorway and Shamshad Khan (2014) have shown that HIV prevention interventions follow established networks of people who identify as members of these key populations or rather construct an identity out of epidemiological categories like MSM. In other words, sexuality exceeds specific categorizations of identities, orientations, and practices of the general population, and many do not identify as belonging to these categories. One night in 2016 in Patna, I returned from the field quite late and was informed by the guesthouse attendant that a government official was waiting for me. I became a bit worried as I went up to the room, where I greeted a young man. He settled in a chair and asked me a few questions about my research and my background, then proceeded to tell me how he was still in love with his older brother's male friend. He described how they had had a passionate affair when they were young and unmarried and concluded by saying: "He got married, and I don't know how to ask him whether he still desires to have sex with me. He might think something is wrong with me because I am still thinking and wanting those activities that we did in our youth when we were young and single." The fact that the government official did not use the language of MSM or gay rights, or that this individual did not organize his desire and sexuality in terms of the hetero/homo binary, reveals the limits of the currency of global health's "vulnerable population" categories as defined through sexuality. Furthermore, the programmatic binaries of "key" and "general" populations render the bodies of sexual minorities who do identify as part of "key population" more vulnerable in the clinic.

CONCLUSION

Understanding the ordinary urgencies and crises faced by the poor would require aggregating the populations separated according to various diseases and concerns in interventions and state policy. HIV is not the sole threat to health and futurity, yet a diagnosis of HIV can make apparent the fragility of living. HIV has what Adia Benton has called a distorting effect (2015). While the people connected to the clinics I worked in are able to manage other, more pressing problems such as procuring food, medicines, and repairs by borrowing from kin, finding intermittent work, and relying on government help, these tasks are harder when living with HIV and insecure health systems. The drug shortages due to inefficient supply chains, the shrinking funds, and the austerity measures enacted by the state do not make HIV a "manageable chronic condition"—chronic conditions are not particularly manageable for the poor in India. A majority of my hijra friends in Orissa died of AIDS-related complications between my first visit to do fieldwork in 2008 and my last visit in 2019. Their deaths took a very specific form of withdrawing from life on learning their diagnosis. They were counseled and put on ART but, as I have indicated, problems with the supply of medication and the ideas of gender and sexuality that accompanied them in the clinics made their adherence to treatment precarious. A few years of intermittent treatment, violence from kin, or abjection and despair meted out to hijras by the world often make them give up ART altogether. They moved out of their homes to escape the violence of families complaining about their care, started living like beggars near shrines, temples, cremation grounds, or public spaces like the railway station. This gradual withdrawal from social life to die is made familiar, broadly available, and acceptable through the history of asceticism in South Asia known as *samadhi maran* (Laidlaw 2005). Hijras would claim this way of exiting life and their claim would be honored by both family members and the HIV counselors of the district.

The reason why the young blood donor committed suicide and hijras walk away from ART is found precisely in the gap between the temporalities of the public health epidemic and the individual ill body, between the state's (and state actors like Dr. A and Dr. T) hegemonic discourses about HIV and everyday life as actually negotiated under immediate constraints of poverty. On the face of it the narrative of positive living heralds the end of the HIV crisis, but this narrative effaces an even larger crisis that surrounds it—that of poverty. The question of crafting a life, living, and maintaining a livelihood in the context of poverty is occluded by focusing on "ending" a single disease. A closer look at the notion of "crisis" reveals it to be a Trojan horse, created through the large infrastructure brought into being by the biosociality of HIV. Hence claims of the "end of crisis" and slogans like "Undetectable =

Untransmissible" imply the dismantling of the political communities that the crisis did forge, as Murray argues (see chapter 7 in this book). HIV interventions pin the value of health onto one disease, where the definition of health is narrowly defined through biological values. The temporality of HIV discourse projects a fantasy of the future as a stable ground that noncompliant subjects will miss out on. But life for the HIV+ poor in India is lived in the everyday, and the future is crafted by stitching one ordinary day to another. Health is of no value if it cannot be transacted and used for opportunities, including immigrating for a better job, as the young man who committed suicide aspired to do.

NOTES

1. I question the validity of high risk in this chapter because the category has highlighted sexuality that falls outside heteronormativity as "risky" (i.e., more likely to cause illness and/or death) at the expense of highlighting the context of poverty. I argue that poverty fundamentally alters the relationship between identity, sexuality, and truth.

2. The Global Fund to Fight AIDS, Tuberculosis and Malaria, often abbreviated as the Global Fund, is an international organization that arranges financing for resources necessary to manage pandemics of AIDS, tuberculosis, and malaria. It was established in 2002 and remains one of the most important actors in the global assemblage of HIV prevention, control, and treatment.

3. For another example of how the HIV+ population is pressed into profit through extractive capitalism by the pharmaceutical industry seeking to measure drug-drug effects, see Thiongane and Graham's chapter in this book.

4. This figure was taken from *Procurement Manual for NACP-III* (2007, 14) that is made available by the Government of India and can be accessed at http://naco.gov.in/procurement-manual-nacp-iii. All Government of India publications meant for knowledge dissemination are in the public domain.

5. At the time of writing (early 2021) it has not been possible to obtain follow-up information on the Indian government's funding plans due to the COVID-19 pandemic. Informal conversations with some participants indicate there are still shortages of ARTs and HIV testing problems have been exacerbated by the COVID-19 pandemic, alongside ongoing legal battles against patents filed for new drugs and formulations such as cabotegravir.

6. In fact, shrinking global health funds led the Indian government in 2014 to whittle down NACO from a separate department under the Ministry of Health and Family Welfare to a program absorbed under the National Health Mission.

7. I am hesitant to use the phrase "unsanitary citizens" as defined by Briggs and Briggs (2003) to describe the profiling of patients for several reasons: First, the phrase refers to the state's essentializing, racist understanding of the poor, but race is not a significant category in South Asia. Second, and relatedly, the actions of the health

care providers show that they would not agree that the poor were undeserving of care and citizenship. In other words, the absence of race in South Asia illustrates how pathologies of poverty are contextually specific.

8. Geary makes a similar argument when he points out that HIV is generalized in the African American population, yet the focus is on sexuality rather than race.

REFERENCES

Benoist, Jocelyn. 2010. *Concepts*. Paris: Cerf.

Benton, Adia. 2015. *HIV Exceptionalism: Development through Disease in Sierra Leone*. Minneapolis: University of Minnesota Press.

Bersani, Leo. 1987. "Is the Rectum a Grave?" *October* 43 (Winter): 197–222.

Bhat, Ramesh. 1996. "Regulating the Private Health Care Sector: The Case of the Indian Consumer Protection Act." *Health Policy and Planning* 11, no. 3: 265–79.

Bhuyan, Anoo. 2018. "A Year Since Stock-Outs, India Continues Slow Roll-Out of Child Friendly HIV Drugs." *Wire*, September 17. https://thewire.in/health/india-child-friendly-hiv-drug-slow-roll-out.

Birn, Anne-Emanuelle. 2014. "Philanthrocapitalism, Past and Present: The Rockefeller Foundation, the Gates Foundation, and the Setting(s) of the International/Global Health Agenda." *Hypothesis* 12, no. 1: 1–27

Briggs, Charles L., and Clara Mantini-Briggs. 2003. *Stories in the Time of Cholera: Racial Profiling during a Medical Nightmare*. Berkeley and Los Angeles: University of California Press.

Chevrier, Claudyne, Shamshad Khan, Sushena Reza-Paul, and Robert Lorway. 2016. "'No One Was There to Care for Us': Ashodaya Samithi's Community-Led Care and Support for People Living with HIV in Mysore, India." *Global Public Health* 11, no. 4: 423–36.

Cohen, Cathy J. 1997. "Punks, Bulldaggers, and Welfare Queens: The Radical Potential of Queer Politics?" *GLQ: A Journal of Lesbian and Gay Studies* 3, no. 4: 437–65.

Das, Veena. 2020. *Textures of the Ordinary: Doing Anthropology after Wittgenstein*. New York: Fordham University Press.

Das, Veena, and Ranendra K. Das. 2007. "How the Body Speaks: Illness and the Lifeworld among the Urban Poor." In *Subjectivity: Ethnographic Investigations*, edited by Joao Biehl, Byron Good, and Arthur Kleinman, 66–97. Berkeley: University of California Press.

Dean, Tim. 2015. "Mediated Intimacies: Raw Sex, Truvada, and the Biopolitics of Chemoprophylaxis." *Sexualities* 18, no. 1/2: 224–46.

Dreze, Jean, and Amartya Sen. 1990. *Hunger and Public Action*. Oxford, UK: Clarendon Press.

Engelmann, Lukas, and Janina Kehr. 2015. "Double Trouble: Towards an Epistemology of Co-infection." *Medicine, Anthropology, Theory* 2, no. 1: 1–31.

Foucault, Michel. 1980. "The Politics of Health in the Eighteenth Century." In *Power/Knowledge: Selected Interviews and Other Writings, 1972–1977*, edited by Colin Gordon, 166–86. New York: Pantheon.

———. 1991. "Politics and the Study of Discourse." In *The Foucault Effect: Studies in Governmentality,* edited by Graham Burchell, Colin Gordon, and Peter Miller, 53–72. Chicago: University of Chicago Press.

Geary, Adam. 2014. *Antiblack Racism and the AIDS Epidemic: State Intimacies*. New York: Springer.

Goffman, Erving. 1978. *The Presentation of Self in Everyday Life*. Harmondsworth, UK: Penguin.

Hegde, B. M. N.d. *Prophetic Thoughts and Articles on Health and Disease Body and Mind.* Vol. 1. Tamil Nadu: TAG-VHS Diabetes Research Centre.

——— 2011. "What We Need Is Not the Will to Believe but the Will to Find Out." *Indian Academy of Clinical Medicine Journal* 12, no. 2: 101.

———. 2012. "Nutritional Immune Deficiency Syndrome." *Moneylife News and Views in Your Interest,* January 17. https://www.moneylife.in/article/nutritional-immune-deficiency-syndrome/22997.html.

Jain, Dipika, and Rachel Stephens. 2008. *The Struggle for Access to Treatment for HIV/AIDS in India*. New Delhi: Human Rights Law Network.

Laidlaw, James. "A life worth leaving: Fasting to Death as Telos of a Jain Religious Life." *Economy and Society* 34, no. 2 (2005): 178–199.

Lorway, Robert, and Shamshad Khan. 2014. "Reassembling Epidemiology: Mapping, Monitoring and Making-Up People in the Context of HIV Prevention in India." *Social Science and Medicine* 112 (July): 51–62.

Mahajan, Manjari. 2008. "The Politics of Public Health Emergencies: AIDS Epidemics in India and South Africa." PhD diss., Cornell University.

———. 2018. "Philanthropy and the Nation-State in Global Health: The Gates Foundation in India." *Global Public Health* 13, no. 10: 1357–68.

Ministry of Health and Family Welfare, Government of India. 2016. *Annual Report 2015–16*. http://naco.gov.in/sites/default/files/Annual%20Report%202015-16.pdf.

———. 2007. *Procurement Manual for NACP-III*. http://naco.gov.in/procurement-manual-nacp-iii.

Nichter, Mark. 2020 "India's National TB Programme: The Struggle for Innovation and Control." In *Understanding Tuberculosis and Its Control: Anthropological and Ethnographic Approaches*, edited by Helen Macdonald and Ian Harper, 185–205. New York: Routledge.

Outlook Web Bureau. 2018. Donor who Attempted Suicide after his HIV Positive Blood Infected Pregnant Woman, Dies. *Outlook*, December 30. https://www.outlookindia.com/website/story/india-news-donor-who-attempted-suicide-after-his-hiv-positive-blood-infected-pregnant-woman-dies/322635

Pilgrim, Nanlesta, Nrupa Jani, Sanyukta Mathur, Catherine Kahabuka, Vaibhav Saria, Neema Makyao, Lou Apicella, and Julie Pulerwitz. 2018. "Provider Perspectives on PrEP for Adolescent Girls and Young Women in Tanzania: The Role of Provider Biases and Quality of Care." *PLoS One* 13, no. 4: e0196280.

President's Emergency Plan for AIDS Relief [PEPFAR] India. 2017. *Strategic Technical Alignment for Results (STAR) Process, Country Operational Plan, Strategic Direction Summary*. https://www.state.gov/wp-content/uploads/2019/08/India-15.pdf.

Press Trust of India. 2018a. "Pregnant Woman Tests HIV+ from Tainted Blood, Donor Attempts Suicide." *Hindustan Times*, December 27. https://www.hindustantimes.com/india-news/pregnant-woman-tests-hiv-from-tainted-blood-donor-attempts-suicide/story-0CdmlekLV4Tu2WogQOiBpM.html.

———. 2018b. "Teen Donor Attempts Suicide after Infecting Pregnant Woman with HIV." NDTV.com, December 28. https://www.ndtv.com/tamil-nadu-news/tamil-nadu-blood-donor-attempts-suicide-after-infecting-pregnant-woman-with-hiv-in-virudhunagar-1968938.

Lalitha, N. 2014. "Regulatory Standards in Pharmaceuticals and Consumers: Missing Links." In *Globalization and Standards*, 143–63. New Delhi: Springer.

Millard, Colin, Abhay B. Kadam, Rushikesh Mahajan, Allyson M. Pollock, and Petra Brhlikova. 2018. "Availability of Brands of Six Essential Medicines in 124 Pharmacies in Maharashtra." *Journal of Global Health* 8, no. 1: 1–12.

Nattrass, Nicoli. 2007. *Mortal Combat: AIDS Denialism and the Struggle for Antiretrovirals in South Africa*. Durban: University of KwaZulu-Natal Press.

Reuters. 2014. "India: Delayed ART Procurement Saw 150,000 PLHIV at Risk of Missing Treatment." Avert.com, October 15. https://www.avert.org/news/india-delayed-art-procurement-saw-150000-plhiv-risk-missing-treatment.

Saria, Vaibhav. 2015a. "The Pregnant Hijra." In *Living and Dying in the Contemporary World: A Compendium*, edited by Veena Das, 83–99. Berkeley: University of California Press. 83–99.

———. 2015b. "To be Some Other Name: The Naming Games that Hijras Play." *South Asia Multidisciplinary Academic Journal* 12: 1–14. https://doi.org/10.4000/samaj.3992

Srinivasan, S., T. Srikrishna, and A. Phadke. 2013. "Drug Price Control Order 2013: As Good as a Leaky Bucket." *Economic and Political Weekly* 48, no. 26/27:10–12.

Sundar, S. 2018. "Pregnant Woman Tests Positive for HIV after Blood Transfusion in Tamil Nadu." *Hindu*, December 26. https://www.thehindu.com/news/national/tamil-nadu/pregnant-woman-tests-positive-for-hiv-after-blood-transfusion-in-tamil-nadu/article25828885.ece.

World Bank. 2013. Restructuring Paper on a Proposed Project: Restructuring of National AIDS Control Support Project. http://documents.worldbank.org/curated/en/224511561348287037/text/Disclosable-Restructuring-Paper-National-AIDS-Control-Support-Project-P130299.txt.

Chapter 2

Governing HIV+ Subjectivities in Post-2011 Egypt

Wesam Hassan

I swear you won't find an AIDS patient in Egypt anymore. I swear you won't find a Hepatitis C patient anymore. We won't import drugs anymore.

—Spokesperson for the Egyptian Armed Forces at a national press conference, February 23, 2014[1]

In this chapter, I analyze an event, the announcement of a device that would allegedly cure HIV and AIDS, in order to illustrate an aspect of the biopolitics of governing HIV and AIDS in Egypt.[2] I present an ethnographic account that represents the responses of my interlocutors, people who are living with HIV, regarding the announced device and its clinical trials. My aim is to portray how my interlocutors engaged with governmental claims of discovering a cure for HIV and AIDS during a period of political, economic, and social unrest in the aftermath of the 2011 Egyptian revolution.[3]

In February 2014, in one of the political events that followed the 2011 revolution, the Egyptian Armed Forces' medical team announced two medical devices. Allegedly, one of the devices could detect HIV and AIDS and hepatitis C, and the other could cure HIV and AIDS and hepatitis C. The latter was called the "Complete Cure Device." At the televised press conference cited in the epigraph above, the Armed Forces announced that they had discovered the device that cures HIV in 2006, but they did not announce it at the time in order to protect their "nation's pride invention" from international pharmaceutical companies. The two devices were endorsed by state officials, including the interim president (Adly Mansour) and the minister of defense,

General Abdel Fattah El Sisi (who has been the Egyptian president since 2014), both of whom were sitting in the front row of attendees.

The Egyptian Medical Syndicate strictly opposed the device and the propaganda surrounding it. The Complete Cure Device was subsequently scientifically criticized and proven ineffective. In January 2015, an Egyptian lawyer filed a lawsuit against the army officials and the medical team who announced, promoted, and participated in the clinical trials for the devices.[4] To date, no significant developments have taken place in relation to the lawsuit.

This announcement of a nation's claim to have found a cure for HIV/AIDS, as well as how it was received and taken up by various interlocutors, led me to ask the following questions: How did HIV+ Egyptian people perceive the "Complete Cure Device" and situate it within the overall social, political, and economic spheres of their everyday lives? How did they consider the announcement of the device: Was the announcement of a medical device that cures HIV/AIDS an accountable political commitment to more care and treatment for them as people living with HIV or to curbing HIV and AIDS in Egypt, or was it something else entirely? Additionally, how did they relate this device to the public debates about HIV and AIDS in the Egyptian streets, the Egyptian media, and ultimately the Egyptian state and its mode of governance?

In analyzing this event and the subsequent conversations about it, I argue that there is an analogy between the human body in a state of weakened immunity after contracting HIV and an enfeebled "body politic" that was manifested in the Egyptian governmental institutions, which were confused after the 2011 revolution. I argue that this analogy between a physical bodily state and the political state of a country contributes to a better understanding of "the interconnectedness of human and national entities" (Biehl, Good, and Kleinman 2007, 8) and of how to navigate bodies and systems in turbulent times.

The analogy between a weakened human body (due to contracting HIV) and a weakened state of national institutions is intended to situate the affected bodies and institutions in the larger scheme of events in Egypt after 2011. This analogy also demonstrates how a medical pathology can be utilized to gain popularity in the political realm by challenging the boundaries between medical, social, and political fields. I am concerned with the ethico-political question of making HIV and AIDS "visible" and acknowledged in the eyes of the public through the propaganda around the Complete Cure Device. The Egyptian military's announcement of the device instrumentalized the language of scientific innovation within the nationalistic discourse supporting the military and its prospects in governing Egypt post-2011. Therefore, situating the device's announcement within the global quest to end the AIDS epidemic allows us to examine the mechanisms through which the global goal of "ending AIDS"[5] is being translated by nation-states.

The February 2014 announcement was not the first time that HIV/AIDS cures and remedies had been announced and promoted by a national government. The governments of Gambia, Iran, and South Africa also announced having found a cure for HIV/AIDS (Fassin 2007, Amon 2008). However, while Egypt is a low-prevalence country where HIV/AIDS is officially claimed to affect less than 0.1% of the population (Khattab 2010, National AIDS Program 2019), the announcement of the device led to the introduction of the disease as part of the everyday rhetoric, humor, and conversations of Egyptians, who generally deny, stigmatize, and "other" HIV/AIDS as a "foreign" disease. For example, reference to the announcement of a "CC device" was an inside joke that many Egyptians used in conversations. "CC" refers to the first letters of "Complete Cure" and also to Sisi (the current Egyptian president, Abdel Fattah El Sisi), who had attended the press conference as the Minister of Defense. The device was also called the "Kofta device" by some people and media outlets, because of a speech that former general Ibrahim Abdelatti,[6] who appeared to be the main inventor of the device, delivered at the conference. General Abdelatti used the word "Kofta device" (meat skewers) as a metaphor to explain how the device would be used to cure HIV, saying "The device will be able to extract HIV from the blood of the patient, and we can take the HIV and make *Kofta* out of it and give the blood back to the patient for nourishment."

Following this announcement, most of the national and international media channels renamed the device as the "Kofta device" or the "Kofta joke." Thus, General Abdelatti's attempt to simplify the explanation of the mechanism and the efficiency of the device for the Egyptian public backfired. Ironically, in popular Egyptian language and everyday slang, "Kofta" usually signifies a person's inefficient or nonsensical actions or sayings. The media and popular responses to the "CC device" and the "Kofta device" were Egyptians' utilization of humor and dark comedy as a mode of resistance.

ENCOUNTERING THE DEVICE

I conducted ethnographic fieldwork in Greater Cairo in Spring 2015, with five mothers who were living with HIV. They were all in their mid-30s, had been living with HIV for more than five years at that time,[7] and came from the working class and lived in poor urban settings in Greater Cairo. Two of the mothers were volunteers who provided support to women who were newly diagnosed with HIV. None of the mothers had a job with a permanent employment contract, and hence they had neither social nor health insurance as a basic employment right.

At the beginning of my fieldwork, I had a conversation with an Egyptian social worker who counseled individuals who were newly diagnosed with HIV. He said that he used a metaphor that describes the body's immune system as an army that defends the entire body against pathogens. When I asked him how the introduction of the Complete Cure Device affected his work and what his stance on the issue was, he said:

> When explaining how immunity works in the body, we use a metaphor that describes the immune system as if it were the body's army and HIV its enemy. I think they understand me better when I use this metaphor, and it also goes well with the country's current political discussions and events. After the announcement of the device, we were confused, and we didn't know what to tell the people who came to consult with us looking for affirmation. People living with HIV and with HCV were checking with us whether it was true that our Armed Forces had discovered the cure. The situation was vague, and the country was highly polarized. If we responded that it was not true, some people would respond that we were not faithful to our army and that the army would not declare such an achievement unless they were certain. Any feedback from our side would be "politically" translated into being with or against the Armed Forces. The truth is that we remained discreet and cautious about our position on the announced HIV/AIDS cure until the propaganda around it faded away. Eventually, everyone knew it was a fraud. There were already HCV medications and people began their treatment regimen, but there was no cure for HIV, as had been announced. (Social worker, Spring 2015)

Emily Martin (1995) has argued that this image of the immune system as an army defending the body has been replaced by an image of the body as a mutable and constantly changing field that is adaptable and flexible rather than a static one that needs to be defended. However, the social worker's statement indicates that the perception of the immune system as an army that protects the body is still prevalent in HIV and AIDS discourses in Egypt. The army–immunity metaphor resonated with the political events of Egypt at the time I was conducting my research, and consequently, what constitutes immunity was contextualized between the biological, the political, and the imagined.[8]

I was interested in examining how my interlocutors perceived the introduction of the device. The responses varied. Some of my interlocutors had hoped for and believed that a cure had been found, while others had denounced the device altogether. Yet others stated that the announced monthly allowance for joining the clinical trials had motivated them to consider participating in the device's clinical trial.

Maha, Amal, and Sama are fictional names for three of my interlocutors who had encounters with the device. Maha participated in the device's first clinical trial and spent three months in the Cairo-based *Homi'yat Abaseya* hospital (fever hospital) where the trials took place. This hospital is also one of the sites where HIV medications are disseminated monthly, free of charge, to people living with HIV. During my initial conversation with Maha, she said, "I can tell you the necessary information about my HIV status. I have been to many HIV-related groups and events. I know the questions that people usually ask me." Her voice was monotonous and tired. However, once we began the conversation about the device, Maha's voice gained more rhythm, and she became more dynamic. She had learned about the device from a poster advertising the need for participants for the clinical trials, and she also knew about the call from officials in the National AIDS Program before it was announced to the public. Maha said:

> Did you know that I was one of the people who tried the device? Before the conference, they gathered us and said, "You are cured of AIDS, and we will announce the device to the public." I was convinced that I was cured. My high hopes and trust in our Armed Forces made me volunteer for the first clinical trial of the device. I told myself, you have nothing to lose by trying the device. If it worked, I would be cured. I left my 3-year-old son with my aunt and my sister, who took care of him. I stayed in the hospital three months for the clinical trial. I witnessed all these men in military suits and all this secrecy, which gave me a grand feeling: that I was participating in a high-level national achievement. This was after the revolution, with positive speeches and aspirations for the new Egypt. Everything seemed possible at the beginning. (Maha, personal interview, Spring 2015)

The announcement of the device as a new scientific discovery animated Maha's nationalistic ideals. Maha's hopes of finding a cure for her medical pathology intertwined with her hopes for her country to achieve an unprecedented scientific breakthrough such as finding a cure for HIV and AIDS. At that time, nationalistic sentiments and the discussions about the new Egypt were driving the public atmosphere after the 2011 revolution. The presence of all these military suits, as Maha described, amplified her sense that she was part of a national breakthrough for her own good and the good of her country.

In another meeting with Maha, I asked: "How did the time pass in those hospital rooms?" Maha preferred to illustrate her journey since she entered the gates of the *Homi'yat* Hospital, to participate in the trials. She described how she felt about the daily routine in the hospital room:

> We gathered in the hospital's garden waiting for each of us to meet the main person behind the device, Dr. Ibrahim Abdelatti. I found out later that he is

> not a real licensed doctor. He used to claim that he treated people with herbal medicine. All of us who went through the clinical trials were living with HIV. When it was my turn to meet Dr. Abdelatti, he asked me how I became infected with the virus and how long I had been living with it. I told him that I was married, that my husband had passed away from the virus, and that I have a child. I was accepted as one of the people who would participate in the clinical trial. In the beginning, when I was admitted, I had a room in the *Homi'yat* hospital, where there were mostly military doctors and soldiers around me. They said that those rooms were rented from the management of the hospital. I stopped my HIV medication for the trial period, as requested, and was only allowed to eat certain food that they provided. No meat at all. Every day we had our sessions by getting connected to the device. I lay down on a bed next to that big device, with the needles inserted in my neck, and all of my blood would go through the device and then return to my body. For me, the device looked like the ones used for renal dialysis in cases of renal failure, which I had seen before in hospitals. I was feverish and exhausted after those device sessions. Dr. Abdelatti would give us daily pills in a small brown glass container with the words "*Allah Al shafi*" ["God is the healer"] written on them. There was no medical label for those pills and no description of what they were made of, as you would see for pills that you get from pharmacies. Every day, he would ask us how we were doing, and he confirmed that we were getting better as he examined our blood tests, and that the HIV virus was being eliminated from our blood. Deep inside, I didn't like seeing him; he did not smile and was very gloomy. (Maha, Spring 2015)

Sitting next to the device reminded Maha of her fragile body and her unstable immune system, which she tries to manage to avoid relapses. At the start of the trials, she was equipped with her hope for a cure along with a certain amount of trust that her disease was now a national issue, and she would be cared for by the state. Maha's trust would diminish as time passed in her clinical trials, and her doubts about the effectiveness of the device would grow. She hoped to see more "white coats," referring to civilian medical doctors, around her. She affirmed that most of the medical doctors sounded as if they were part of the military medical team.

Reflecting on her experience, Maha observed:

> Now, whenever I remember how I was convinced that I got better and my body was being cured of the virus, I feel betrayed. I was relieved at the end of the clinical trial to be reunited with my child. Who knows, I could have died in those three months. I was suffocating in that room for three months, not allowed to leave the hospital, and my psychological state was very bad. (Maha, Spring 2015)

Maha spent the three months of the clinical trials inside the hospital and was not allowed to go outside. She described her feelings as swaying between hope and despair, trust and doubts, and she feared thinking about leaving the trial and returning to her home. After all, the Armed Forces had made the exceptional move of positioning the cure of HIV and AIDS as a national priority and as an attainable promise, thus inciting debates in the Egyptian streets about a disease that was stigmatized in the public discourse. "Maybe if the Armed Forces had found a cure, the stigma around HIV would have diminished," Maha contemplated. The "exceptional" deployment of HIV and AIDS by the authorities at that particular time exemplifies Aiwha Ong's (2006) argument about neoliberal modes of governance. Neoliberalism is tied not only to economic models, Ong states, but also to modes of governance in which the states can adopt exceptional practices to accumulate political power and "reengineer" the political space (Ong 2006, 220).

Amal was another interlocutor who had different views about the device. She was a *niqabi* (face-covered) woman and had an outgoing friendly manner. She was able to compensate for her hidden facial expressions with her captivating voice and eyes that bristled with strength and liveliness to the point that I forgot she was wearing a *Niqap*. As we spoke, she uncovered her face and shared that she had been suspicious about the lack of clarity about the entire process of the device from the outset:

> I felt that it was a fraud. It was a gut feeling. Maybe this thought resulted from what I have witnessed during the years since 2011 and all of the political events and empty promises of a better future. When I heard about the device, I was skeptical. The main reason was that I was sure that if anything went wrong during this treatment that had been announced by the army, no one would be held accountable, sued, or judged [*Yet'haseb*]. How can you put a military person on trial because of the failure of an AIDS cure? You can't put a military suit [*Badla meeri*] on trial. Moreover, I have three children, so how could I leave them for three months and be confined in a hospital room for the clinical trial? I know that my HIV medication is helping me to move on with my life and provide care for my children. I hope for a cure; however, I made peace with the idea that there is none. It took me some time to reach this conclusion. I won't spoil it and dream of an unattainable cure. Now I wake up every day praying for the health that will allow me to get through the day for the sake of my children. I renew my prayers every morning. One day at a time. Ultimately, I look forward to the day when I will see my children well-educated, married, and living their own lives. (Amal, Spring 2015)

Amal's attitude toward the entire device phenomenon, her character, and her takes on life reminded me of Deleuze when he stated, "There is no need to fear or hope, but only to look for new weapons" (Deleuze 1992, 3). However, Deleuze does not explain what these new weapons are. In the context of my research, my interlocutors' negotiations or bargaining techniques with different authorities were their weapons. Their will to live was tangible, and their techniques were constantly mutating. One of their techniques was their own spiritual practices and deep faith in God and Islamic traditions. Another technique was adopting a philosophy of life, such as thinking about or looking for life "one day at a time," in order to manage their hopes and dreams. These negotiations represented internal dialogues with HIV along with their external dialogues with medical, social, and legal authorities.

Sama, my third interlocutor, looked younger than her age, with a smiling face and youthful open attitude. She had been hoping for an opportunity to participate in the device trials primarily because of her financial need for the thousand Egyptian pounds that were offered as a monthly allowance to the trials' participants. She arranged for a family member to take care of her almost eight-year-old child. Sama recalled most vividly the authoritarian and militarized manner in which officials conducted interviews with individuals who came to participate in the clinical trials:

> I waited so long in the hospital's garden—it was a warm day, and we were tired. Finally, we were able to enter, and I heard a nurse telling a young person standing with us in the line: "You look gay; don't tell Dr. Abdelatti that you got HIV from sleeping with men; he will not let you enter the clinical trial." When I entered the interview room and stood in front of Dr. Abdelatti, I was stressed. His looks were not encouraging, and he rarely raised his face from the papers he was looking at. He asked me about my age and then immediately asked, "How did you get infected with HIV?" I told him it was directly from my husband, as I am married. Dr. Abdelatti then asked me how my husband got infected, and I answered that he has an addiction problem and injects drugs. Dr. Abdelatti immediately told me, "Go tell your husband to get clean and stop drugs and then come together with you for another trial." I was disappointed and felt humiliated. I knew what happened to some of the people who were waiting with me . . . [they] were treated more horribly than I was. For example, he asked one of the women "How did you get the virus?" and she said, "I don't know." He dismissed her, saying that she was a prostitute who slept with many people and didn't know where she got the virus. Another woman was wearing a *Nikab* covering her face. Dr. Abdelatti asked her to remove it, and she refused. He dismissed her as well, saying that he wouldn't let "ghost-like" people participate in the trials for the device. It was as if he was holding a ruler, a morality ruler (*mastarra*), and using it to measure the ethics and morals of the people entering the trials! He was dismissing anyone he thought was immoral! As if some of us deserve to be cured and others don't! In the end, I am happy that I was not

> selected, especially since I found out later that some people died from complications and opportunistic diseases during those trials. They had to stop taking their HIV medications for the three months of the trials. In the end, their families can't prove that they died from the clinical trials because they had AIDS, which is considered a death sentence, anyhow. (Sama, Spring 2015)

This quotation from Sama makes it evident that moral judgment and prejudice were strategies that were used to decide who deserved to be cured. Sama's comment reveals how a certain moral judgment by authorities would decide who would be involved in the clinical trials of the device. In the turbulent times after the 2011 revolution, morality was used as an apparatus to accumulate political power by gaining social support and building social capital via media outlets and state's institutional declarations. Speeches were made about the importance of maintaining conservative Egyptian ideals and guarding the country's moral identity so that it would be able to transition peacefully to stability. Issues around the presence of Western agendas that affected the stability and security of Egypt, such as the spread of the Western ideals of individualism, personal freedom, and autonomy, were widely used by the Egyptian media and government as tools for suggesting a conspiracy against Egypt.

Sama's comments portrayed Dr. Abdelatti's, and therefore the Egyptian state's, ethico-moral position on people living with HIV. Dr. Abdelatti's comments reinforced the concept of "self-responsibility" regarding how one was infected or protected. His attitude conveyed his understanding of what is considered an appropriate "social order" and how to "other" those who don't abide by it. My research interlocutors were aware of the ways in which HIV-positive people are stigmatized compared to people who live with hepatitis C. Sama reflected on this issue: "It is a burden to think every time before answering the question, how did you get AIDS? They do not ask people with Hepatitis C how they got it. I have no choice but to answer. If I don't answer, they judge that I got the virus from a shameful forbidden practice and not in an innocent way, like from my husband or through a blood transfusion."

In their narratives, my interlocutors disclosed their struggles with biopolitical technologies of governing HIV and their exposition and critique of those technologies. They also affirmed that HIV and AIDS comprise one part of a multitude of intersecting factors in a set of social, economic, and legal inequalities that render some groups of people more vulnerable than others (Oraby and Abdel-Tawab 2016, 9). Their vulnerability comes from their internalized social belief that there is a collective moral code and that by being infected by and living with HIV, they have pushed the limits and even destroyed the imagined and practiced social and moral codes of the society in one way or another. The "moral calculus" (Farmer 1992, 109) related to

HIV and AIDS was deployed when selecting people who would go through the clinical trials, for example, by selecting only "innocent victims" when deciding who could and couldn't participate in the device's clinical trials (here "innocent" is meant in the sense of contracting HIV from a socially acceptable source, such as a husband or blood transfusion).

WHAT CONSTITUTES "THE POLITICAL"?

What was the impact of my interlocutors' experiences with the Complete Cure Device? Were they now more cynical and critical about modes of governing HIV and AIDS and its spaces of care and treatment? Did they still have hope and optimism for a change to come in the ways in which people living with HIV and AIDS were being addressed and cared for? Were they able to grow beyond any confinement caused by a disease or an authoritarian regime?

In probing these questions, I found that my interlocutors had been deeply influenced by their HIV+ status and by the incident of the complete cure device. Amal shared her realization that they (HIV+ people) are sometimes used to get funding for different projects related to HIV in the development sector. She said that the image and the presence of an HIV+ person and the announcement of a device that would cure HIV are examples of manipulating HIV+ people, especially with the emphasis on "innocent" ways of getting infected with HIV and stereotyping people as being innocent or not.

On the other hand, Sama expressed that her philosophy in life had changed since the 2011 revolution, and later on her encounter with the device. She lamented that she lost her brother in one of the events after 2011, which was more traumatic for her than her HIV diagnosis. Sama said: "I became more proactive about what kind of life I want to live and prioritized what matters first. It was my son and my health. I divorced my husband and looked for a job. I learned how to stand on my feet again after multiple defeats."

Maha became more vocal in expressing her needs and was in a continuous process of reflection, asking herself: What was disrupted in her life by the announcement of the device and the clinical trials? The answer was that her acceptance of her HIV+ status and her daily routine that she had struggled to structure had been disrupted. Her HIV treatment regimen—the strong recommendation of adhering to HIV treatments—had also been disrupted by the clinical trial. Her acceptance and her newly figured-out routine required the greatest of efforts to enable her to take care of her son. Yet her participation in the clinical trials gave her the false hope, that an HIV cure had been found, which collided with her endeavor to assemble a life in which she accepted her HIV status and the need for her daily medication.[9]

Maha, Sama, and Amal agreed that as time passed, they overcame the initial shock and learned how to live with HIV. They gained more understanding about their bodies and their bodies' needs in the process of living with HIV. They struggled to establish new routines to move on with their lives. This was a continuous process of negotiation and bargaining with their own bodies and with different authorities in their lives. It was a journey of continuous becoming and transcending from one phase or structure to another. This particular journey was hindered and disrupted by the device with its false hopes and failed promises.

HIV and AIDS are modern pathologies that are shaped by multiple forms and hierarchies of power and that in turn shape the subjectivities of people affected by them. In this entangled reality, individuals like my research interlocutors grapple with authorities like the Egyptian state and its biomedical interventions. In this context, any public or personal struggle turns into a political struggle, because "there is no face in which the political doesn't appear. Power is everywhere" (Navaro-Yashin, 2002, 3). The political here has no site, that is, "it is not confined to the boundaries of its rationalized institutional and discursive forms" (Navaro-Yashin 2002, 2).

The collective responses of my interlocutors highlighted that biopower is not limited to only the state's polices and governmental bodies, but also applies to the circulation of power through different hierarchies, entities, and discourses that create the political realm. Sama, Amal, and Maha demonstrated techniques of resisting, escaping, and/or negotiating with state authorities, without them conceptualizing their daily struggle as a political one. What constitutes the political here is the interplay between two forces: the force of authority and the force of resistance, whether in subtle, everyday acts or as a direct confrontation. Hence, subjects who negotiate possibilities of altering realities within the dominant control and discipline are considered political (Badiou 2008).

CONCLUSION

I began my ethnographic research with a Foucauldian theorization focused on examining whether the biopolitical governing HIV and AIDS would lead to the subjugation of the people living with HIV (Nkomo and Long 2014). After conducting the fieldwork, I realized that Deleuze's argument of the "primacy of desire over power" (Biehl and Locke 2010, 317) would better reflect on the conatus within my interlocutors, as they negotiated the tangled web of authorities and resisted the structured subjugation process. I consider their conatus, in Spinozian terms, as the effort to "venture beyond the negative aspects of the present" (Garcia 2017, 113). My interlocutors' conatus was their desire to negotiate, analyze, live, and try to care for themselves and their loved ones. They were in a continuous state of creating new routines that evolved through the different phases of their lives, the multiple "subjectivities" they performed, and their encounters with "new" knowledge and claims about HIV/AIDS. This continuous state of "becoming" provided them with the resilience and plasticity to accept and negotiate life's precariousness and uncertainty (Biehl and Locke 2017, X). They negotiated, and continue to negotiate, the dominant political, social, and medical structures surrounding them while performing their roles as mothers, workers, and women of particular class positions and cultural backgrounds. However, it is not only the people who have the virus in their blood who live with uncertainties and precarity. Key emotions and experiences that they expressed, such as uncertainty, fear, stress, solitude, discrimination, helplessness, being judged, and questioning the concept of "free will," are expressed in our everydayness and mirrored in others.

Engaging with my interlocutors has highlighted for me the fragility of public health models and national strategic health plans. Notions of public good or neoliberal economics center self-responsibility at the core of being infected with HIV and pave the way to "exceptional modes of governing" (Ong 2006, 3) through a pathology, in order to orchestrate the political arena. The analysis I have presented in this chapter is not intended to offer a comprehensive background on HIV and AIDS systems of care and support in Egypt. Rather, it provides documentation of one of the alleged cures for HIV, adding to the plethora of literature on the anthropology of HIV and AIDS, particularly in a site that is depicted by statistics showing low HIV prevalence numbers. It also depicts how the bodies of people living with HIV (Comaroff 2007) have been utilized and entrapped in the body politic of state authorities (Nkomo and Long 2014) in turbulent times after 2011.

In conclusion, I was inspired by the stories of the mothers I met while doing this ethnography.[10] As they shared their narratives, with all their differences and resemblances and their lamented and cheerful moments, they sounded to me as if they were a choir chanting together their collective laments. *Cantus Lamentus*, a music composition by Dhafer Youssef, has moved me to imagine these mothers singing their sorrows in an ensemble. The narratives they composed are woven together to transcend their own individual stories, providing a background of melancholic melodies for the everyday events of their precarious living, with all of its random, chaotic yet lively, and pulsating encounters. Their stories point to their continuous acts of mediating the political, the social, and the medical circumstances within which they were situated while living with HIV in Egypt. The stories carry vibes of agony and melancholy as these women figured out, on a daily basis, how to survive the demands of their roles as mothers, workers, women, and Egyptians. However, their faith was tangible in their continuous acts of negotiating the consequences of appalling life events. There was cathartic power in the telling of their stories, as if they were singing out their sorrows. Their "song" provides room to contemplate, relate to, and reflect on the art of living itself. That is what music does to the listener, and that is what happened to me while encountering the stories they shared, for which I am grateful.

NOTES

1. https://www.theguardian.com/world/2014/feb/28/egypt-unveil-device-detects-cures-aids

2. I extend my gratitude to my interlocutors who have shared their experiences and stories with me. I am immensely thankful to Dr. David Murray for his many helpful and detailed comments, insights, and editorial expertise on the chapter. I also extend my appreciative thanks to Dr. Adia Benton who provided astute reflections and comments on the early version of this chapter when I presented it as a conference paper in the annual American Anthropological Association Meetings in 2019. This text is part of my MA research and dissertation at the American University of Cairo, in which I greatly benefited from the wisdom and mentorship of Dr. Martina Rieker, Dr. Hanan Sabea, Dr. Reem Saad, and Dr. Malak Rouchdy. All the names of my interlocutors have been changed to pseudonyms.

3. The 2011 Egyptian revolution was a popular uprising against corruption, police brutality, and the social and economic injustice of President Hosni Mubarak's regime, which ruled Egypt for over 30 years. The uprising forced Mubarak from his power as a president. In the aftermath of 2011, Egypt had a period of social, political, and economic unrest. Egypt was ruled by the Supreme Council of the Armed Forces from February 2011 till June 2012. On June 30, 2012, Mohamed Morsi, who was affiliated with the Muslim Brotherhood, was elected and sworn in as the Egyptian president. Later, Morsi was overthrown by a military coup and the current president Mohamed El Sisi was sworn into presidency on June 8, 2014.

4. http://www.dailynewsegypt.com/2015/01/05/lawsuit-targets-army-officials-claiming-hiv-hepatitis-c-cure/

5. Ending the HIV/AIDS epidemic is a global goal of the 2015 United Nations (UN) Sustainable Development Goals. This goal requires a political commitment, along with other economic and social commitments, and cooperation from UN member states. The goal of ending AIDS was announced and coupled with clear and precise numeric indicators that need to be achieved by 2030. In 2014, UNAIDS developed a fast-track policy aiming to (1) mainstream testing in order to ensure that 90% of the people who are HIV+ know their HIV status, (2) ensure that treatment is provided for 90% of HIV+ people, and (3) ensure that 90% of the people being treated would have an undetectable viral load. To further the global commitment to end AIDS, a high-level UN meeting on AIDS was held in June 2016, to focus on reinvigorating the commitment of UN

member states to ending the AIDS epidemic. The emergence of the "End of AIDS" policy is an important part of the context of this chapter, as it relates to the global political goal of ending AIDS (other economic aspects of ending AIDS manifested in the pharmaceutical companies' strategies, the commitment of the Global Fund for AIDS, TB, and malaria, and their policies are not mentioned here).

6. http://www.akhbarak.net/articles, accessed on March 12, 2015. Although General Abdelatti is not a licensed medical doctor, he uses herbal medicine as a holistic practitioner and claims that he can treat people for cancer and autoimmune diseases, among others. A lawsuit based on accusations that he was not a trained, licensed medical doctor has been filed against him. Although he is a civilian, he was given the rank of general for unknown reasons. He announced the CC device as his invention and said that it was endorsed by the Armed Forces. Dr. Gamal Sheiha, who is an internal medicine expert specializing in liver disease and hepatitis C, said that he didn't know Abdelatti and didn't work with him on the CC device. Dr. Sheiha is the primary inventor of the C-Fast device, which detects hepatitis C virus in infected persons, and its patent is registered under his name.

7. An important criterion for my ethnographic research was to conduct it with mothers who were not newly diagnosed with HIV. This comes from my conviction that the trauma of recent diagnosis needs specialized personnel who are trained in psychosocial support. I didn't have specialized training for providing counseling. Hence, I worked with mothers who already had more than five years to listen to and understand their newly figured routines and learned life philosophies that they acquired from living with HIV in Egypt.

8. Biologically speaking, the T cells, part of the white blood cells that constitute the immune system, have to remember the pathogen to be able to react to it. Thus, they are given the name "memory T cells." When the T cells cannot remember the pathogen, the body fails to recover by itself and needs outside help, such as medical treatment. Therefore, the work of immunity is initially a work of memory. However, my interlocutors didn't recognize it as such. They all assimilated the work of immunity to the army metaphor.

9. The moment of rupture caused by receiving a positive HIV diagnosis creates a state of psychological, emotional, and social disturbance in which people living with HIV fear what is coming next. I call this a "moment of rupture" because at the moment of being diagnosed, my interlocutors had not yet configured new realities or routines. They suddenly faced the reality of a precarious life, which turned their imagined future into a distant past. For many of them, panic arose when they were forced to choose between holding on to their previous techniques of survival and configuring new techniques to assemble a new life with a fragile immune system.

10. For more details about the ethnographic study, please see Hassan (2016).

REFERENCES

Amon, Joseph J. 2008. "Dangerous Medicines: Unproven AIDS Cures and Counterfeit Antiretroviral Drugs." *Globalization and Health* 4, no. 1: 5.

Badiou, Alain. 2008. "The Communist Hypothesis." *New Left Review*, 49: 29–42.

Biehl, João, Byron Good, and Arthur Kleinman. 2007. *Subjectivity: Ethnographic Investigations*. Berkley, CA: University of California Press.

Biehl, João, and Peter Locke. 2017. *Unfinished: The Anthropology of Becoming*. Durham, NC: Duke University Press.

Biehl, João, and Peter Locke. 2010. "Deleuze and the Anthropology of Becoming." *Current Anthropology*, 51, no. 3: 317–51.

Bloch, Ernst, and Neville Plaice. 1986. *The Principle of Hope*. Vol. 3. Cambridge, MA: MIT Press.

Comaroff, Jean. 2007. "Beyond Bare Life: AIDS, (Bio) Politics, and the Neoliberal Order." *Public Culture* 19, no. 1: 197–219.

Garcia, Angela. 2017. "Heaven." In *Unfinished: The Anthropology of Becoming*, edited by Biehl João and Locke Peter, 111–30. Durham, NC: Duke University Press.

Farmer, Paul. 1992. *AIDS and Accusation: Haiti and the Geography of Blame*. Berkeley, CA: University of California Press.

Fassin, Didier. 2007. "When Bodies Remember: Experiences and Politics of AIDS in South Africa." Berkeley, CA: University of California Press.

Hassan, Wesam. 2016. "Cantus Lamentus: Navigating HIV Positive Mothers Subjectivities in Egypt Post 2011." Master's thesis, The American University in Cairo. http://dar.aucegypt.edu/bitstream/handle/10526/4637/Wesam%20A.%20Hassan-Thesis-Fall%202015.pdf?sequence=1.

Khattab, H. 2010. "The Agony of AIDS: A Qualitative Study on the Experience of AIDS in Egypt." Cairo: Egyptian Society for Population Studies and Reproductive Health (ESPSRH).

Khattab, H. 2014. "Living with AIDS: Suffering and Courage." Cairo: Egyptian Society for Population Studies and Reproductive Health (ESPSRH).

Martin, Emily. 1995. "Flexible Bodies: Health and Work in an Age of Systems." *Ecologist* 25, no. 6: 221–26.

Navaro-Yashin, Yael. 2002. *Faces of the State: Secularism and Public Life in Turkey*. Princeton: Princeton University Press.

Nkomo, Nkoma, and Carol Long. 2014. "Governmentality, Subjectivity and AIDS." *Subjectivity* 7, 411–31. https://doi.org/10.1057/sub.2014.16

Ong, Aihwa. 2006. *Neoliberalism as Exception: Mutations in Citizenships and Sovereignty*. Durham, NC: Duke University Press.

Oraby, Doaa and Nahla G. Abdel-Tawab. 2016. *Understanding married Women's Vulnerability to HIV Infection in Egypt: An Exploratory Study*. Cairo: Population Council.

Youssef, Dhafer. "Cantus Lamentus Dhafer Youssef." YouTube video, 3:47. October 4, 2009. https://www.youtube.com/watch?v=XA805hs8CT0

Chapter 3

Disclosure and Responsibility

Children Living with HIV in Uganda

Colleen Walsh Lang

Eleven-year-old Violet,[1] Counselor Helen and I are seated inside a shipping container repurposed to serve as the counselor's office. Violet has never met the counselor before and maintains her gaze fixed upon the floor. I'm seated behind Violet, to observe, but not interfere with the intimate discussion which is about to unfold. After the standard greetings, the counselor asks Violet if she knows why she takes medications every day. Violent points to her scars. The remnants of the itchy rash caused by HIV are still visible on her arms and legs.

Counselor Helen responds, "yes, these things on your skin used to pain you; but you came [here] and they gave you medicine the things [lesions] left you. Isn't it so?"

Violet nods in reply.

"And yet, you are still taking medicine" the counselor continues, "do you know why?"

Violet sits quietly.

"Have you ever heard of the virus [pause] which brings Slim?"[2] Counselor Helen asks.

Violet nods, and when asked explains what her mother told her about it: "Maama said that the little thing of Slim pains badly." Violet's mother has passed away from AIDS, and it was her death which prompted Violet's testing and diagnosis; however, it is not clear whether Violet knows that her mother died because of AIDS. The "little thing" which Violet refers to is the virus, HIV. When Violet first arrived at the treatment center she was in very poor health, but over the past six months, she has recovered, and will be returning home to live with her grandparents soon. She also had nightmares about her mother's death when she first arrived but has been sleeping well for several months.

"Mmm [yes]" Counselor Helen replies, "it pains badly if you don't take the medicines. . . . But, when you take medicine, it doesn't do what? It doesn't pain.

But, when he/she doesn't take medicine it does what? People who don't take medicine it pains badly. It is true, what she [your mother] told you."

"Nnn [un hu]" Violet nods, still keeping her eyes downcast.

"Now, for you, do you know why you take medicine?" probes the counselor.

"No" Violet responds.

"Would you like to know why you take the medicines?" she asks.

"Nnn [yes]" Violet nods.

Counselor Violet goes on, "If I disclose to you, will it make you feel good? Will you continue to take the medications well?"

"Nnn [yes]," Violet nods.

Counselor Helen then explains that Violet has tested positive for HIV, and that she most likely got the virus from her mother, because, "Children get it from Maama during birth or breastfeeding, but not because they want, but it just happens [accidentally]." She emphasizes the importance of medication adherence and quizzes Violet on her medication names, times, and doses. She attempts to address and dispel common myths about HIV being a death sentence or about transmission via casual contact.

Violet responds mostly with nods, yes's and no's, avoiding direct eye contact, and Counselor Helen does most of the talking, despite her efforts to ask open-ended questions. At one-point Violet begins to cry quietly, and the counselor reiterates her reassurances that if Violet takes her medications "very well" she will be healthy, and that although the virus will always be in her blood, the skin lesions will not return. She tells Violet that having the virus is not her fault, and she should not feel ashamed. However, at the end of the conversation, once Violet has stopped crying and appears to be feeling better, she instructs Violet that "this is our secret" and that she should not tell other people about her having HIV.

It's a lot to take in in a single session, but Counselor Hellen tells Violet she will visit her before Violet returns home, and that Violet should come by with her (grand)parents whenever she comes to get her medications from the clinic.

This vignette is typical of a disclosure session for the children that I worked with. My research focuses on the experiences of children living with HIV in Uganda. The children I worked with were accessing HIV care through an NGO which I refer to as Baaliro. Through my research, I gained insights into children's experiences living with HIV in the "post-crisis" era, especially how they came to learn about HIV and how they understand the meaning of their own seropositive status in their lives. The "post-crisis" era is one in which, ostensibly, people infected with HIV, adults and children alike, have access to free antiretroviral drugs (ARVs)—the medications which keep HIV from taking over a patient's immune system. In the "post-crisis" era, children living with HIV can live full healthy lives, but that life hinges upon adherence to ARVs. However, the seemingly simple act of taking medications every day is not so simple as notions of responsibility and ever-present stigma interact to obstruct disclosure to children. Children, meanwhile, may understand more than they say, and, I argue, their silence and reluctance to talk about HIV speaks volumes about their knowledge of the gravity of the disease they are facing.

Access to ARVs has given HIV the potential to be a chronic manageable illness; however, countless scholars have described the difficulties adults face in adhering to even the simplest ARV regimens, including medication side effects, the need to take medications with food, difficulties accessing mediations, and the psychological fatigue of taking medications daily (e.g., Kalofonos 2010; Van Dyk 2010). Patients who "fail" to take their medication properly are easily labeled as "noncompliant" and "irresponsible," and historically these arguments were used to delay access to ARVs in low-income countries. However, issues of noncompliance are not unique to HIV nor to the developing world (Chesney, Morin, and Sherr 2000; Mehta, Moore, and Graham 1997; Rintamaki et al. 2006).

Meanwhile, children face additional challenges, in that they are often dependent on adults to access medical care and, as I describe below, may not understand why they are taking medications (Campbell et al. 2012; Schenk et al. 2014). Importantly, dependence should not be conflated with a lack of agency, as children constantly work to understand and influence their world (Bluebond-Langner and Korbin 2007; James and James 2008; Lancy 2012). HIV research is not unique in its tendency to overlook the experiences of children, and in this chapter, I make a small step in redressing this oversight.

In this chapter, I present children as active agents living with HIV. All the children I worked with had access to ARVs, though nearly all presented to medical care in crisis—they were diagnosed with HIV after having become very ill, sometimes more than once. In sharing their stories, I show that anti-HIV stigma remains a powerful force in their lives, shaping the process of disclosure, the experience of treatment, and children's understanding of their disease. I begin by briefly describing access to ARVs in Uganda and show how, ironically, as the elimination of mother-to-child transmission of HIV becomes more of a reality, those children living with HIV become signs of failure and sources of stigma, rather than symbols of success. I then introduce Baaliro—the site of my research and a residential treatment/rehabilitation center for children living with HIV. Children present to Baaliro in crisis, receive treatment and rehabilitation, and are ultimately reintegrated into their home communities. I discuss how, despite staff's recognition of the importance of disclosure for improving children's adherence to daily medications, staff ultimately spend more time searching for a responsible caregiver[3] who will ensure medication adherence. Paralleling the neoliberal ideologies of

Western funders, the local staff emphasize and demand individual (caregiver) responsibility for treatment success. Meanwhile, children may understand more than they directly express, and their reluctance to discuss HIV explicitly may be due to their knowledge of HIV stigma, and their attempts to keep it at bay. Finally, through the story of one of the children (Peter), I demonstrate that the definition of a responsible caregiver can be a slippery concept and that identifying one can be an even more complex and contested process. These challenges can result in responsibility being shifted to the child himself, through the means of disclosure. Overall, claiming that we have entered a "post-crisis" era for HIV fails to acknowledge ongoing crises for these children—in being diagnosed, in identifying caregivers, in understanding and accepting their own diagnosis, and in living with HIV every day.

The arguments presented in this chapter are based on 16 months of ethnographic fieldwork. I lived at Baaliro for 11 of those months from July 2014 to June 2015. My primary research method was participant observation. I strove to achieve the "least-adult role" in my interactions with children and to focus on their perspectives (Mandell 1988). In my role as an observer I was granted access to witness six disclosure conversations—when a counselor told a child he/she had HIV, ostensibly for the first time. I requested and was granted oral permission to record these sessions.[4] While I was living at Baaliro, 24 children spent a month or more living at the center and nine children stayed for one to three weeks. I also interacted with four children, who had previously been treated at Baaliro and now volunteered at least weekly at the center, and 74 children who I visited with briefly either during visits to their home/school (57 children) or when they came to Baaliro for appointments (17 children). Children's ages ranged from 8 months to 25 years, but the majority were 8–14 years old.

UGANDA: MOVING TOWARD A "POST-CRISIS" ERA WITH ARVS

Uganda has long been upheld as a model country for its early national response to HIV/AIDS, and for being the first African country (if not the first country globally) to report a decline in adult HIV prevalence (Parkhurst 2005; Kleinman et al. 2011). HIV messaging initially focused on prevention, with ABCs (abstain, be faithful, condomize) being the pillar of messaging. While the posters may have changed since the advent of ARVs, the emphasis on prevention and individual responsibility remains.

The dramatic and rapid rollout of ARVs in the early 2000s changed the landscape of HIV care in Uganda and offered the possibility of (new) life to those infected with the virus (Whyte 2014). However, the rollout was uneven in many ways including eligibility criteria and access to treatment (see figure 3.1). Initially efforts targeted pregnant women for the prevention of mother-to-child transmission (PMTCT), much later rolling out ARVs to children themselves. Furthermore, one of the main consequences of increasing access to treatment has been a reemphasis on individual responsibility—to be tested and to take treatment "properly" if one tests positive. This messaging is especially heightened for women of reproductive age.

In 2011, UNAIDS introduced the *Global Plan towards the Elimination of New HIV Infections among Children by 2015*. While not utilized in this initial document, the approach would eventually be shortened to the acronym eMTCT (*elimination* of mother-to-child transmission [of HIV]). With this new emphasis on *elimination*, Uganda reported that "a remarkable reduction in new infections among children was achieved; from 27,660 in 2011; 15,411 in 2012, and 9,629 in 2013" (Uganda AIDS Commission 2014, viii, 7). While reducing the number of new infections in children is overwhelmingly a positive thing, having elimination as the goal makes those children who are infected into signs of failure. The failure is multitiered, at the level

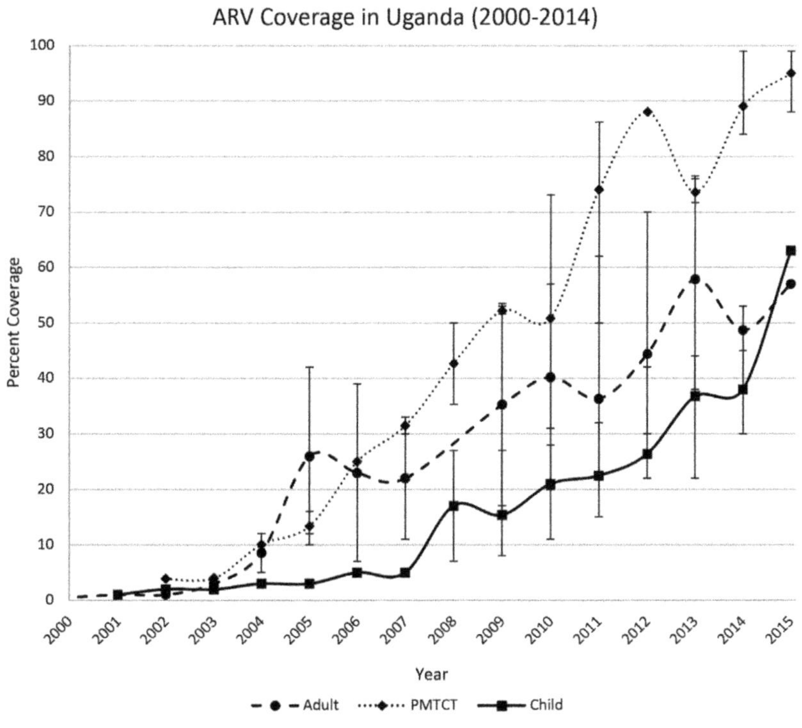

Figure 3.1 ARV Coverage in Uganda (2000–2014). *Source*: Graph created by Colleen Walsh Lang.[5]

of mothers, health care workers, the community, and even the nation as a whole; however, mothers bear the brunt of the stigma and shame. Several studies looking at barriers to getting children enrolled in ART and to disclosure of a child's HIV status have shown that stigma and shame often delay both the initiation of pediatric treatment and disclosure (Abadía-Barrero and LaRusso 2006; Boender et al. 2012; Cree et al. 2004; Kajubi, Whyte, et al. 2014; Lowenthal, Jibril, et al. 2014; Ostrom et al. 2006; Schenk et al. 2014; Vreeman et al. 2013). This burden can, ironically, be especially strong in communities where PMTCT messaging is widespread, because mothers feel more responsible for having not protected their children from infection (Class 2014).

Given the prevalence of HIV-prevention messaging, perhaps it is not surprising that despite Uganda's status as a model country for its commitment to fighting AIDS, stigma and misinformation remain persistent problems. As stated in the Uganda AIDS Commission's 2015 report, "There are still several socio-cultural factors that are *increasing* HIV stigmatization" (emphasis added) (Uganda AIDS Commission 2015, 50). While children themselves may be pitied rather than blamed for being infected, they and their caregivers (especially if the mother is surviving) can experience "cascade stigma" if the child's status is revealed (Deacon and Stephney 2007; Murphy, Roberts, and Hoffman 2002; Schenk et al. 2014). In Mozambique, Deena Class (2014) found that HIV-prevention messages which focus on sexual fidelity and PMTCT enhance the stigma of mothers who have HIV+ children by implying that they must be promiscuous (to have been infected in the first place) and irresponsible (because responsible mothers can prevent their children from becoming infected), regardless of the fact that numerous researchers have demonstrated that monogamy and marriage are actually risk factors for HIV (Hirsch et al. 2010; Mkandawire-Valhmu et al. 2013; Tolan 2005). Didier Fassin (2013) takes this analysis one step further arguing that the construction of children as innocent victims worthy of assistance hinges upon the portrayal of others (adults) as negligent and unworthy. In Uganda, the desire to protect children from stigma is frequently cited as a reason to delay disclosure, which itself leads to problems with adherence (Fallon 2014; Kajubi, Whyte, et al. 2014). Even simply attending a known HIV clinic can lead to disclosure of a child's HIV status, thus making caregivers reluctant to initiate treatment for HIV-infected children (Schenk et al. 2014).

BAALIRO: THE MEANING OF REHABILITATION

Within this context, of increasing, but still uneven access to HIV treatment and highly prevalent stigma, Baaliro was built. The idea for Baaliro came from collaboration between a Swiss NGO, founded by a former volunteer, and the staff at a locally founded HIV clinic. The HIV clinic was founded in 1998 by a group of five Ugandans (one of whom is now Baaliro's program director) as a health care organization dedicated to improving the lives of people infected and affected by HIV. The clinic has received funding from a variety of national and international donors, including the Stephen Lewis Foundation, USAID, Irish AID, Elton John, the Inter-Religious Council of Uganda, and individual donors. The clinic offers not only medical services but also social outreach, youth programming, counseling, and economic support to people living with HIV. It is an independent NGO, and not part of the government health care system, but does receive ARVs from the Ugandan government.

In 2002, a 16-year-old Swiss volunteer came to work at an orphanage and school near the HIV clinic. He returned for several years, and ultimately founded a NGO, financed by Swiss donors, which supports several non-HIV-related programs such as children's education and caregiver's economic empowerment. While volunteering at the orphanage he witnessed the severe problems that children faced when "aging-out" of the classical orphanage system. Children had lost ties to their families and had no social/community support once they turned 18. They often struggled not only with surviving financially but also with substance abuse and mental health issues. He became convinced of the importance of children maintaining ties with and (ideally) being raised by their own family members. During his time in Uganda he also accompanied children to their clinic visits at the HIV clinic and discussed the challenges the staff was facing including struggling to care for HIV-infected children who came from rural villages. They had witnessed many HIV+ children deteriorate and die after being discharged from the local hospital. The children lived too far away, and their families did not have the resources to return when the children became ill and/or to return to pick up medication refills. The idea of Baaliro was born from these conversations—to provide a longer-term, but still temporary, treatment center to allow children to fully medically stabilize and to provide access to medications and monitor adherence once the children had been "reintegrated" home. The volunteer ultimately raised funds from individual Swiss donors to build Baaliro in 2008 and continues to fund the program through his NGO. Baaliro is run entirely by Ugandan staff in close partnership with the neighboring HIV clinic, and Baaliro staff report to the Swiss NGO several times a year.[6]

Baaliro offers a unique treatment model in which children are admitted to a residential treatment facility for medical stabilization with the ultimate goal of having them "reintegrated" (the term used by Baaliro) to their home communities to be raised by family members. Children normally presented to Baaliro with advanced HIV infection and stayed at the facility for 2–20 months, with a median stay of six months. In an effort to normalize living with HIV, while at the facility, children were expected to participate in housework and attend a nearby school as much as their health allowed. Staff at the center emphasized treating the children "like any other child" rather than seeing them as "sick" children. Baaliro employees followed up with reintegrated children, providing school fees and adherence support.

At the most basic level, rehabilitation required simply getting children to swallow their medications and to eat their food. Baaliro tracked children's rehabilitation by monitoring their lab results and measuring their physical bodies. In practice, however, the tasks of taking medications and feeding were not always so simple, and the metrics used to track rehabilitation told only part of the story. In addition to these metrics, staff paid attention to several aspects of children's responses to treatment, including the ease with which children took their medications, their patterns of food refusal, and any side effects the child reported. HIV and nutritional rehabilitation were not separate but intertwined. As staff often said, "*eddagala lyagala mmere*" [medications [i.e., ARVs] need/want food]. Staff also took into consideration children's attitudes and behaviors as well as whether their caregivers were "responsible"[7]—all of which were predictors of successful reintegration.

If forced to identify a single criterion for determining if a child qualified for care at Baaliro or was ready for reintegration, the staff would point to the CD4 count,[8] because it provided a numerical indicator of immune system function which in turn served as a proxy for the response of the virus to the ARVs. Although a CD4 count is the most important laboratory indicator of immune system function and the strongest predictor of HIV progression (UNAIDS 2015), it does not directly measure the amount of HIV virus or its response to medications. So, although CD4 count is actually not the best metric for assessing a patient's response to ARVs, the clinic did not have access to viral load testing and thus used CD4 count as a proxy.

The CD4 count was so important that even once a child had cleared all of his/her opportunistic infections, Baaliro could delay reintegrating him/her because of his/her CD4 count. Baaliro did not have a set cutoff for children's CD4 count, but always became concerned if it dropped below 200 cells/mm^3, and a count below 50 cells/mm^3 was itself cause for immediate (re)admission to Baaliro. CD4 counts improved very slowly and therefore were only tested at most every three months. Among reintegrated children, low CD4 counts were one of the most common reasons for a child to rebound to the center. A low CD4 count meant that treatment was not working—either because of poor adherence (i.e., the child was not taking his/her ARVs), viral resistance to the medications (often assumed to be a consequence of poor adherence), or both.[9] This marker of response to treatment has very concrete consequences, as a low CD4 count corresponds with susceptibility to infection, and thus staff understandably wanted to keep children at the center until their immune systems had recovered as much as possible, or get them back into treatment if their CD4 count had dropped.

However, preparing children for reintegration was about more than just this blood test. Staff also monitored how easily children took their medications. Staff emphasized that the long-term success of children's rehabilitation hinged upon them continuing to take their medications once they returned home. While at Baaliro staff utilized a variety of strategies with children who were reluctant to take their medications, ranging from positive encouragement and offering treats to threats of hospitalization and, as a last resort, holding a child down to forcibly give him/her the medications. Physical restraint was highly ineffective and undesirable, and I only witnessed it being used a handful of times, typically with children under the age of four who were deemed too young to understand the importance of taking medications. Overall, the staff emphasized using positive strategies to get children to take their medications without a struggle. They explained that they needed children to continue taking their medications once they were reintegrated, and caregivers could not be expected to put forth such herculean efforts to get a child to take medications every day.

The head nurse closely watched the facial expressions of children when they took their medications and later (out of the earshot of children) discussed her interpretations with me. She was attentive to children grimacing or wrinkling their noses as signs that they did not want to take the medications and as she explained to me, "many of them, they fear taking the medications." Since this indicated that a child would likely stop taking the medications once he/she returned home, such facial expressions signaled to her that she needed to counsel the child.

Counseling, however, did not consist of scheduled sessions and did not require lengthy discussions. In fact, it did not even necessarily involve disclosure of the child's HIV status, but rather consisted of frequently encouraging the child to take medications. For example, in the case of a particularly recalcitrant six-year-old girl, Sister Sally repeatedly asked her throughout the day, "are you going to take your medications tonight?" Over time the girl agreed to take her medications, and after a few weeks of this, she would willingly swallow her pills without discussion. Sister Sally also regularly reminded children that they took, "*eddagala lya'bulamu*" [medications for life/health].[10] This double meaning—both that children will take medication for the rest of their lives, and that taking medication was necessary for their health/lives—was not lost on the children. Overall, the staff took what they described as a "soft approach" to changing children's attitudes toward medications. It was important that children become used to taking medications and accept medications without argument or struggle because once they had been reintegrated, staff explained, caregivers could not be expected to spend much time or effort getting children to take their medications. To give the children the best chance at adherence, and therefore life, they needed to take their medications easily.

Staff at Baaliro often talked to me about the importance of disclosing children's HIV status to them, and, in fact, attributed the difficulties they observed with poor adherence, especially among adolescents, to a lack of early disclosure. However, they rarely mentioned HIV at Baaliro, despite the opportunity to do so at twice daily medication times. Instead children repeatedly heard the refrain "medications are for life" and were only told that if they didn't take them, they would die. Staff discussed HIV more openly among adults and at youth workshops;[11] however, they cited two factors which inhibited their discussions with younger children: (1) parental refusal of disclosure and (2) lack of resources to explain HIV to younger children. While at first it may seem surprising that disclosure was not part of rehabilitation, many scholars have described the reluctance of caregivers and clinicians to disclose children's HIV status to them (Kajubi, Whyte, et al. 2014; Lowenthal, Bakeera-Kitaka, et al. 2014; Midtbø et al. 2012a; Ostrom et al. 2006; Szelag 2011; Vreeman et al. 2013 and many more). Most of this reluctance hinges upon a desire to protect children from stigma as well as a fear that children will disclose their status to peers or community members, and thus expose caregivers to cascade stigma.

Nonetheless, staff at Baaliro agreed that children *should* be disclosed to at an earlier age, and in recent years had started having disclosure discussions with a counselor for some children prior to reintegration. The hope was that by disclosing to children earlier, they themselves could take responsibility for taking their medications, especially in cases where the staff was concerned that a caregiver was "irresponsible." Unfortunately, these disclosure discussions were a one-time event and took place with a counselor from the affiliated HIV clinic who, though trained in discussing HIV with children and pediatric counseling, the children had never met before.

Ideally, disclosure is more than a one-time event (Abadía-Barrero and LaRusso 2006; Brada 2013; Kajubi, Bagger, et al. 2014; Lowenthal, Jibril, et al. 2014; Midtbø et al. 2012b; Pinzón-Iregui, Beck-Sagué, and Malow 2013). Especially for children, whose cognitive capabilities are constantly developing, disclosure should be an ongoing discussion. Many have shown that a single disclosure event does not give children adequate time to understand, ask questions, and process the meaning and significance of having HIV. Also, by only speaking about HIV once, children receive the unspoken message that it's not okay to talk about HIV openly. As I discuss in more detail below, children clearly receive this unspoken message and are reluctant to talk about HIV. Finally, it is better for disclosure to come from someone who the child trusts. The Uganda staff agreed with these ideals; however, the logistics of the social worker's workload as well as her discomfort having disclosure discussions lead to the situation described above.

WHY DO YOU TAKE MEDICATIONS EVERY DAY?

In my research I found that despite having lived at a HIV treatment center for months at a time, only about half of the children named HIV/AIDS as the reason why they took medications daily (see tables 3.1 and 3.2). The main responses children gave to the question "why do you take medications every day?" were "I don't know/I forgot" or to name another illness. Other illnesses named included ulcers, tuberculosis, cough/chest infection, leg/joint pain, syphilis, to prevent malaria, to prevent diarrhea, for deworming, and more generically "because I'm sick."

Table 3.1 Why Do You Take Medicine Every Day?

Why Do You Take Medicine Every Day?	*Number of Children (%)*	*Age in Years Avg (Range)*
HIV/AIDS	35 (56%)	13.9 (8–17)
Never names HIV/AIDS	28 (44%)	10.4 (6–17)

Responses of children when asked, "Why do you take medications every day?" (N=63). HIV/AIDS—Includes English or *Luganda* terms: HIV, AIDS, *mukenenya, sirimu.*
Note: Four children required considerable prompting before naming HIV/AIDS. Researcher only prompted children when certain that staff had recently had a disclosure conversation with them.
Source: Table created by Colleen Walsh Lang, Original data collected by Colleen Walsh Lang.

Table 3.2 Other Reasons Given for Taking Medication

Other Reasons Given for Taking Medications	
Don't know/forgot	18
Names another illness/Generic illness ("I'm sick")	11
General health	7
Refuses to answer	4
Uses HIV-related terms	3
NOT HIV	2

Responses of children who did not name HIV/AIDS as the reason for why they took medications.
Another illness—Ulcers (seen on chest X-ray), TB, *ekifuba* (chest infection/cough), leg/joint paint, syphilis, to prevent malaria/diarrhea, for deworming, "because I'm sick."
General health—*Kuwona* (to heal), because I don't want to die, to stay healthy, *"eddagala lya'bulamu"* [medications for life/health].
HIV terms—(to keep CD4 up, "so the soldiers will fight the insects") [but won't name HIV itself].
Note: Twelve children gave more than one reason for taking medications.
Source: Table created by Colleen Walsh Lang, Original data collected by Colleen Walsh Lang.

Overall children were visibly uncomfortable discussing why they took daily medication. Even after having lived with many of the children for weeks, if not months (recall that 17 children had stayed at Baaliro for greater than one month and five for one to three weeks while I was living there); even though discussions took place in a confidential location; even after multiple visits; and even (in some cases) after I had sat in on the child's disclosure conversation—many of the children were reluctant to discuss why they took medication, and especially reluctant to name HIV/AIDS (whether in English or Luganda). They would look down, fidget, and remain silent or speak in whispers when I broached the topic. Among the six children for whom I was present during their disclosure conversations, when I later asked them if they remembered why they took medications every day, none readily answered my question. Four of them would not name why they took medications even with prompting and two did so only with considerable prompting.

It is difficult to disentangle whether the children truly did not know why they took medications, or if they knew, but were unwilling to name the virus responsible. As exemplified in Violet's disclosure conversation, in one breath children are explicitly told that HIV is nothing to be ashamed of, that it is not their fault, and that they should not be treated differently because of it; and in the next, they are told not to tell anyone (other than "safe" people like doctors, counselors, and caregivers) that they are HIV+. The fact that children were so uncomfortable talking about HIV/AIDS and medications indicates to me that they may have known that they had HIV/AIDS and had internalized the stigma about the virus and were thus reluctant/ashamed to discuss it. In her work with children in Malawi, Hunleth describes the way children avoid naming taboo illnesses such as HIV and tuberculosis, yet know a great deal about these conditions and their treatments (2013). Children's reluctance to name the virus/disease even in a "safe" place and with "safe" people indicates to me that children are aware that HIV is not a "safe" topic. Perhaps they see that caregivers become uncomfortable when talking about HIV. If so, I see this as an example of children's desires to protect both themselves and their caregivers from shame/stigma. This is not a new concept; in the 1970s Bluebond-Langner documented that children as young as three years old were aware that they were dying of cancer, but would not discuss their knowledge with their parents because they did not want to distress them (1978). Children can be more attuned to the needs of and implicit messages sent by the adults around them that we often give them credit for. In the "post-crisis" era of HIV, children may be demonstrating their awareness that being a child living with HIV is shameful, because their infection could have been prevented, by their reluctance to talk about it.

THE IMPORTANCE OF RESPONSIBLE CAREGIVERS

Given that few children could/would talk about having HIV, it is difficult to discuss how they experienced living with HIV. From children's perspectives, the most important factor in their lives was who their caregiver was. This was the person that they would stay with, who would (if they could afford it) buy them shoes and ensure that they had good food to eat. From the staff's perspective, this was also the most important factor in the success of reintegration since this was the person who would ensure that children took their medications. Interestingly, despite how much staff spoke to me about disclosure, they ultimately focused more on finding a responsible caregiver than disclosing a child's status. In fact, disclosing to a child was primarily done only as a last resort if the staff had difficulty identifying a "responsible caregiver."

Baaliro staff frequently pointed to Peter's mother (*Maama*-Peter) as a paradigmatic example of an irresponsible caregiver. Peter was first admitted to Baaliro in June 2012 when he was seven years old. Although he had tested positive for HIV in 2009, he did not start taking ARVs until his admission to Baaliro. He also had not attended school prior to arriving at Baaliro, but while at the center he started in baby nursery (the lowest level class) and was quickly promoted to middle nursery class after only half a year. While at the center, the social worker's reports described Peter as being very interested in schooling, clean and smart,[12] helpful, disciplined, respectful, and overall, well behaved. One staff member declared, "indeed he is a good influence to others," and my own recollection of Peter from the summer of 2012 was that he was a vibrant intelligent child who was a joy to interact with. Peter stayed at the center for nearly 10 months and was reintegrated to his mother's care in March 2013, near the end of the first school term.

Upon reintegration, Peter's mother was given the responsibility of finding and registering him in a school, so that Baaliro could pay for his school fees; however, she never found a school for him to attend. As early as May 2013, the social worker ominously noted in Peter's chart, "the mother is experiencing a lot of social problems which might affect the child's future." For the rest of 2013, *Maama*-Peter changed homes several times and never enrolled Peter in school. In September, the social worker noted that Peter's health had started to deteriorate and identified the fact that Peter lacked a "definitive home location" as the cause of both his poor adherence to ARVs and lack of schooling. By January 2014, Baaliro staff was unable to locate Peter or his mother, and the social worker summarized the situation:

> We have been trying to get in touch with the mother [of Peter] but have failed. [A staff member] went to make inquiries at the [maternal] grandfather's place,[13] but they told him the mother had left the home and went to live with [Peter's]

other grandmother in some village in Buikwe. They haven't heard from her and do not know of her whereabouts. (Case file note, January 2014)

At this point Baaliro staff had not seen Peter for three months. The social worker documented their plan: to find Peter and once found to enroll him in a boarding school and identify another relative to look after him during school holidays, "because the mother is irresponsible and will not look after him well" (case file note, January 2014). In February 2014, *Maama*-Peter brought Peter to Baaliro and reported that he had not been taking ARVs for over two months. The staff informed her of their decision to enroll Peter in boarding school and noted no objection. Later that month, the social worker visited Peter's paternal great-aunt (*Jjajja*-Peter)[14] who lived near the boarding school where Peter was to be enrolled. *Jjajja*-Peter agreed to visit Peter while he was at school and to have him stay with her over the holidays.[15]

Maama-Peter accompanied her son as he was enrolled in the boarding school and a few weeks later she reported that she had checked in on him and he was doing well. However, less than eight months later, when *Maama*-Peter brought Peter to Baaliro in the last week in October 2014 for his medication refill and CD4 count test, the social worker, with her propensity for understatement, said simply "he did not look happy." When the results came back, his CD4 count was only eight and staff determined that urgent action was needed. On November 4, 2014, we made a special hour-and-a-half drive to pick him up from the boarding school and bring him to Baaliro to be readmitted. When we met Peter at school, he looked miserable. In contrast to the vibrant and talkative child I met in 2012, he was sullen and quiet. He seemed small, thin, and frail. He was bony everywhere—his collar bones, hip bones, shoulder blades, and spine were all prominent, along with bony knees and elbows which emphasized the thinness of his limbs. Fungal rings merged together to cover nearly his entire scalp and a silver-dollar sized patch on his right temple seemed ready to take over his eye. This was only the visible fungus, and he continued to suffer from thrush in his mouth and throat for many weeks. As the social worker described it, "the fungal infection has eaten him."

Despite multiple attempts to contact her, the staff was unable to directly inform *Maama*-Peter of their decision to bring Peter back to Baaliro. They told the school's bursar where Peter was going in hopes that when *Maama*-Peter came to check in on him the school would inform her of Peter's whereabouts and she would come to find him at Baaliro, and they continued to attempt to call *Maama*-Peter using the phone number(s) they had on file. They also called Peter's maternal grandfather (who lived near Baaliro), but he said he did not know where *Maama*-Peter was. Somehow, *Maama*-Peter got the word that her child was at Baaliro, and on December 17 (more than a month after Peter had rebounded), she came to the center. However, she only spent one night with her son before leaving. *Maama*-Peter came because she wanted to take Peter to her home for the holidays (Christmas and New Year's), but the staff considered such a request irresponsible, since her home was "deep in the village," far from Baaliro and other medical care. Given Peter's fragile medical condition, they refused her request. Rather than stay at Baaliro with her son, or bring other family members to the center, she left him at Baaliro, and Peter was the only child who did not spend any time over the holidays with his family. *Maama*-Peter next visited her son after the Christmas and New Year's holidays in January 2015 and continued to visit Peter once every one to two months. She would usually stay only a day or two but would wash Peter's clothes before leaving, and at least once she also trimmed his nails and hair. Despite these visits, staff still considered her rude and irresponsible. In addition to her history of failing to find a school for Peter in 2013, they pointed to her lack of a permanent home, her own poor adherence to ARVs,[16] and her desire to take Peter home before she had a permanent place to stay. Also, they pointed out that she was not helpful around Baaliro and that her visits were suspiciously timed with national holidays. The timing of her visits with holidays implied that she came in anticipation of beef or (better yet) chicken being served, and on at least one occasion when she arrived and discovered that only posho and beans were being prepared, she left almost immediately.

At the end of April 2015, the social worker brought Peter to visit *Jjajja*-Peter and learned that when Peter had previously lived with her, he had been taking his medications well and even used to help *Jjajja*-Peter remember to take her ARVs. Apparently, when Peter was with her for the school holiday in August 2014, *Maama*-Peter came and took the boy, which initiated a quarrel between *Jjajja*-Peter, *Maama*-Peter, and Peter's father. *Jjajja*-Peter and Peter's father still had strained relations; however, after the social worker facilitated discussion between them, *Jjajja*-Peter agreed to once again take on the responsibility of caring for Peter when he was reintegrated. This time, the plan was that Peter would live with her full time and attend a nearby day school, since the boarding school had "failed completely." Additionally, Peter's father agreed to assist *Jjajja*-Peter with financial support. The social worker implored Peter's father to visit the boy while he was at Baaliro and assured *Jjajja*-Peter that Baaliro would involve community leaders to ensure that *Maama*-Peter would not take the boy away again without permission. While they reached this agreement in April (between the first and second school terms), Baaliro staff decided to keep Peter at Baaliro until the end of the year both so that they could ensure that his CD4 count was increasing and so that he could complete the school year without changing schools yet again.

Staff also decided to disclose Peter's HIV status to him at this time. Though he was only nine years old and they were not usually disclosing to children that young, they reasoned that if Peter understood why he needed to take medications every day, he might play a more active role in his medical adherence. Peter was intelligent, highly motivated, and at times extremely stubborn. Staff hoped that these traits would make him able to understand what it meant to be HIV+ and keep him motivated to take his medications. But, perhaps most importantly, if Peter had a more "responsible" caregiver, they would not have considered disclosing to a child of his age.

By the time Peter was reintegrated in December 2015, the staff's assessment of responsible guardianship had shifted once again. Neither *Jjajja*-Peter nor Peter's father visited Peter while he was at Baaliro which, according to the social worker, demonstrated "a lack of commitment from that side." Meanwhile, *Maama*-Peter continued to visit Peter every few months, began taking her ARVs consistently, and insisted that she wanted Peter to stay with her. The staff was still concerned about her history of lacking a stable home and of "disappearing," so they "gave the mother strict conditions that she had to live in [a village near Baaliro] and that she has to bring the boy for [ARV] refills, which she agreed upon" (email correspondence with the social worker, September 30, 2016). Both Peter and his mother were doing well, living with Peter's maternal grandfather[17] in a town near Baaliro. Peter was healthy and actively attending school, and *Maama*-Peter was also healthy and was earning money selling charcoal. Baaliro's staff remained cautiously optimistic. They had plans to involve *Maama*-Peter in a microcredit program to improve her economic status, but emphasized that "monitoring at home and counseling is still done so that she can still fulfill her responsibilities over the boy" (email correspondence with the social worker, September 30, 2016).

Peter's case demonstrates why Baaliro staff put such a strong emphasis on identifying a responsible caregiver, that they made considerable efforts to find and communicate with responsible caregivers, and that they constantly reevaluated their assessment of whether or not a caregiver was responsible. This case also helps to complexify the notion of responsibility. It is notable that Peter's HIV status was disclosed prior to him being reintegrated. The staff's concern about finding a responsible caregiver led them to hope that Peter himself, still in early primary school, would quickly come to understand why he needed to take medications and be motivated to take them despite not having a responsible caregiver to support him. Overall, the process of disclosure acted to shift the burden of responsibility onto Peter.

When I interviewed Peter the following year, he initially refused to tell me why he took medications every day. His lab tests indicated that he had been taking his medications as prescribed and he was healthy and doing well in school. According to *Maama*-Peter, he helped her to remember to take her medications as well. It seems unlikely that this bright and witty boy would have forgotten that he and his mother were infected with HIV, and indeed after considerable prompting he named the virus responsible for his being hospitalized twice previously.

CONCLUSION

Overall, though Ugandan children have improved access to ARVs, which are unquestionably lifesaving medications, the stigma and the emphasis on individual responsibility—for prevention of HIV, for adults administering treatment to children, and for children themselves taking medication—remain dominant in lives of children living with HIV. Stigma acts as a major barrier to disclosure of HIV to children, and children's implicit awareness of it hinders continued discussions of HIV with them. The emphasis on individual responsibility, especially for preventing the transmission of HIV to children, places additional burden on caregivers. These children's lives are certainly not "post-crisis."

"Post-crisis" implies postdanger, poststruggle; for a life-threatening illness it's post-the-turning-point when the patient is headed toward recovery rather than death. For the children at Baaliro none of this was true. First, the children at Baaliro were almost all diagnosed through crisis. They came to the center sick with opportunistic infections, some truly at death's door. While the treatment center focused on medical rehabilitation and adherence to ARVs, which can make HIV a chronic manageable (noncrisis) disease, the difficulties of living with HIV did not stop with effective treatment; and children were always at risk of "rebounding" to the center (15% of reintegrated children had to be readmitted to Baaliro for two or more weeks). The danger of HIV and of poor adherence was omnipresent. Despite knowing the benefits of early and frequent disclosure of HIV status for improving children's willingness to take medications, HIV was rarely discussed at Baaliro. Instead, the greatest struggle involved finding responsible caregivers that children could rely on to meet their needs, including helping them take ARVs. At times family members refused to care for HIV-infected children, fearing the stigma of the disease, fearing the virus itself, or both. HIV impacted children's lives daily, yet HIV was rarely if ever discussed openly in front of them. This paradoxical situation made it extremely difficult to directly ascertain children's perspectives on HIV and the impact it had on their lives, but undoubtedly, the effects of the virus were omnipresent.

In this chapter, I have shared pieces of the lives of children infected with HIV in Uganda and of an organization dedicated to helping children recover from and live with HIV. I have shown that stigma remains a strong negative force not only despite, but explicitly *because of* claims that Uganda is "post-crisis" and has "eliminated" mother-to-child transmission of HIV. Children's understanding of their disease is hindered by lack of disclosure and open conversation about HIV, and yet children themselves may understand more than adults realize. Their reluctance to talk about HIV may signify their deeper understanding that HIV is a dangerous topic to be avoided. Meanwhile staff search for responsible caregivers, and if unable to identify them, may disclose to children, thus shifting the responsibility of medication adherence onto children themselves. Given the struggle that these children survive—in being diagnosed, in identifying caregivers, in understanding and accepting their own diagnosis, and in living with HIV every day—it is hard to accept claims that they have entered a "post-crisis" era for HIV.

NOTES

1. All names of individuals and institutions/organizations used throughout this chapter are pseudonyms. As much as possible, identifying factors have been removed.
2. Slim disease (pronounced su-rī-mu) is one of the colloquial terms for AIDS in Uganda.
3. I use the term caregiver rather than parent because the majority of children at Baaliro were not living with a parent. Among the HIV+ children enrolled in Baaliro's program, one or more parents were listed as the primary caregiver only 45% of the time, with grandparents (23%), aunts and uncles (22%), and siblings (4%) making up the remainder of relatives caring for children.
4. This research was also approved by both the institutional review board at Washington University in St. Louis and the Uganda National Council for Science and Technology. Both organizations approved a waiver of written consent for my interactions with and interviews of children and caregivers. As an institution, Baaliro granted preliminary permission for those children staying at the center without a caregiver to participate in my research, and I obtained informed verbal consent from guardians as soon as possible. Children verbally assented to the study.
5. Data was compiled from the sources cited below and included the following reports from Ugandan Governmental Ministries: HIV/AIDS Country Progress Reports (2008, 2010, 2012, 2014, and 2015), the National Strategic Plan for HIV/AIDS (2003–2006, 2007–2012, 2011–2015, and 2015–2020), as well as reports by UNAIDS and UNICEF. When more than one value was provided for a given year, the values from all reports, which provided a value for that year, were averaged. The error bars represent high and low estimates for the year. Coverage estimates were unavailable prior to 2000 and for the following years: children prior to 2001, PMTCT prior to 2002, adults in 2008. Data sources: (UAC 2004, 2007, 2008, 2010, 2012a, 2012b, 2014b, 2015a, 2015b, UNAIDS 2013, 2014b, 2014a, 2015b; UNICEF 2010).
6. For greater discussion of these organizations, see my dissertation (Walsh Lang 2020).

7. For greater discussion of the growing emphasis on responsibilization at Baaliro, see Walsh Lang (2019).

8. A CD4 count is a lab test that measures the number of CD4 T-lymphocytes (CD4 cells) in a sample of blood. A normal range is 500–1,600 cells/mm^3. A count of less than 200 is AIDS defining (aids.gov 2016).

9. See also Betsey Brada (2011) for a discussion of clinicians' preferences for laboratory tests rather than patient reports to measure adherence to ARVs.

10. Whyte and her contributing authors also noted the double entendre of ARVs being medications for life—both life-giving and life-long (2014).

11. Youth workshops were a relatively new innovation at Baaliro. The first workshop occurred during my preliminary fieldwork and was deemed a success, with the hope of having an annual workshop thereafter.

12. Smart here refers to the British usage of neat, clean, or well dressed, rather than the more common American usage of quick-witted or intelligent, though in Peter's case he was both.

13. Peter's maternal grandfather lived near Baaliro, but he refused to take any responsibility for Peter or to allow Peter to stay with him. He was also not always on good terms with *Maama*-Peter.

14. *Jjajja* is typically translated as grandmother; however, it can mean maternal or paternal grandmother, grandfather, great-aunt, or great-uncle, and may even be extended to cousins of that generation.

15. She was apparently not willing to take on the responsibility of having Peter live with her full time, otherwise he would not have been sent to the boarding school.

16. In April 2014, when she visited Peter, *Maama*-Peter was found coughing up blood. She admitted to having stopped taking ARVs two years prior. She was evaluated for TB, but based on a chest X-ray, the doctors declared she did not have TB. She agreed to start taking ARVs again at that time, but her adherence remained poor. She complained of side effects and told my research assistant and me that she would not continue taking the medications once Peter was back in her care.

17. Interestingly, this is the same grandfather they contacted when Peter was brought back to Baaliro in 2014 and who had previously refused to allow Peter to stay with him. Although the grandfather clearly knew when Peter was at Baaliro, he never once visited Peter and refused to allow him to visit for the holidays, despite his proximity to the center.

REFERENCES

Abadía-Barrero, César Ernesto, and Maria D. LaRusso. 2006. "The Disclosure Model versus a Developmental Illness Experience Model for Children and Adolescents Living with HIV/AIDS in São Paulo, Brazil." *AIDS Patient Care and STDs* 20 (1): 36–43. https://doi.org/10.1089/apc.2006.20.36.

aids.gov. 2016. "CD4 Count." July 14, 2016. https://www.aids.gov/hiv-aids-basics/just-diagnosed-with-hiv-aids/understand-your-test-results/cd4-count/.

Bluebond-Langner, Myra. 1978. *The Private Worlds of Dying Children*. Princeton, NJ: Princeton University Press.

Bluebond-Langner, Myra, and Jill E. Korbin. 2007. "Challenges and Opportunities in the Anthropology of Childhoods: An Introduction to 'Children, Childhoods, and Childhood Studies.'" *American Anthropologist* 109 (2): 241–246. https://doi.org/10.1525/aa.2007.109.2.241.

Boender, T. Sonia, Kim C. E. Sigaloff, Joshua Kayiwa, Victor Musiime, Job C. J. Calis, Raph L. Hamers, Lillian Katumba Nakatudde, et al. 2012. "Barriers to Initiation of Pediatric HIV Treatment in Uganda: A Mixed-Method Study." *AIDS Research and Treatment* 2012 (February): e817506. https://doi.org/10.1155/2012/817506.

Brada, Betsey Behr. 2011. "Botswana as a Living Experiment." Ph.D. Dissertation, Chicago, IL: The University of Chicago. http://gradworks.umi.com/34/60/3460154.html.

———. 2013. "How to Do Things to Children with Words: Language, Ritual, and Apocalypse in Pediatric HIV Treatment in Botswana." *American Ethnologist* 40 (3): 437–51. https://doi.org/10.1111/amet.12031.

Campbell, Catherine, Morten Skovdal, Zivai Mupambireyi, Claudius Madanhire, Constance Nyamukapa, and Simon Gregson. 2012. "Building Adherence-Competent Communities: Factors Promoting Children's Adherence to Anti-Retroviral HIV/AIDS Treatment in Rural Zimbabwe." *Health & Place* 18 (2): 123–31. https://doi.org/10.1016/j.healthplace.2011.07.008.

Chesney, Margaret A, Michel Morin, and Lorraine Sherr. 2000. "Adherence to HIV Combination Therapy." *Social Science & Medicine* 50 (11): 1599–605. https://doi.org/10.1016/S0277-9536(99)00468-2.

Class, Deena M. 2014. "Effects of HIV Prevention Messages on Treatment-Seeking and Adherence for HIV-Infected Children in Maputo, Mozambique: A Qualitative Study." *Children and Youth Services Review*, Children and Youth Growing Up with HIV Infection in Sub-Saharan Africa: Implications for Health Service Delivery, 45 (October): 64–73. https://doi.org/10.1016/j.childyouth.2014.03.039.

Cree, Viviene E., Helen Kay, Kay Tisdall, and Jennifer Wallace. 2004. "Stigma and Parental HIV." *Qualitative Social Work* 3 (1): 7–24. https://doi.org/10.1177/1473325004041129.

Deacon, Harriet, and Inez Stephney. 2007. "HIV, Stigma, and Children: A Literature Review." Cape Town, South Africa: HSRC Press. http://www.hsrcpress.ac.za/product.php?productid=2197.

Fallon, Amy. 2014. "ARVs a Bitter Pill to Swallow for Ugandan Children." *Inter Press Service News Agency*, May 7, 2014. http://www.ipsnews.net/2014/05/arvs-bitter-pill-swallow-ugandan-children/.

Fassin, Didier. 2013. "Children as Victims: The Moral Economy of Childhood in the Times of AIDS." In *When People Come First: Critical Studies in Global Health*, edited by João Biehl and Adriana Petryna, 109–32. Princeton, NJ: Princeton University Press.

Hirsch, Jennifer S., Holly Wardlow, Daniel Jordan Smith, Harriet M. Phinney, and Shanti Parikh and Constance A. Nathanson. 2010. *The Secret: Love, Marriage, and HIV*. Nashville, TN: Vanderbilt University Press.

Hunleth, Jean. 2013. "'ARVs' as Sickness and Medicine: Examining Children's Knowledge and Experience in the HIV Era in Urban Zambia." *AIDS Care* 25 (6): 763–66. https://doi.org/10.1080/09540121.2012.748878.

James, Allison, and Adrian L James. 2008. *Key Concepts in Childhood Studies*. Los Angeles, CA; London: SAGE Publications Ltd.

Kajubi, Phoebe, Stine Bagger, Anne R. Katahoire, David Kyaddondo, and Susan R. Whyte. 2014. "Spaces for Talking: Communication Patterns of Children on Antiretroviral Therapy in Uganda." *Children and Youth Services Review*, Children and Youth Growing Up with HIV Infection in Sub-Saharan Africa: Implications for Health Service Delivery, 45 (October): 38–46. https://doi.org/10.1016/j.childyouth.2014.03.036.

Kajubi, Phoebe, Susan Whyte, Simon Muhumuza, David Kyaddondo, and Anne R Katahoire. 2014. "Communication between HIV-Infected Children and Their Caregivers about HIV Medicines: A Cross-Sectional Study in Jinja District, Uganda." *Journal of the International AIDS Society* 17 (1). https://doi.org/10.7448/IAS.17.1.19012.

Kalofonos, Ippolytos Andreas. 2010. "'All I Eat Is ARVs':" *Medical Anthropology Quarterly* 24 (3): 363–80. https://doi.org/10.1111/j.1548-1387.2010.01109.x.

Kleinman, Sarah, Julie Rosenburg Talbot, Julian Harris, and Andrew Ellner. 2011. "Cases in Global Health Delivery: The AIDS Support Organization (TASO) of Uganda." Harvard Business Publishing. https://cb.hbsp.harvard.edu/resources/marketing/docs/GHD008p2.pdf.

Lancy, David F. 2012. "Unmasking Children's Agency." *AnthropoChildren* 1 (2). http://popups.ulg.ac.be/AnthropoChildren/docannexe.php?id=1503.

Lowenthal, Elizabeth D, Sabrina Bakeera-Kitaka, Tafireyi Marukutira, Jennifer Chapman, Kathryn Goldrath, and Rashida A Ferrand. 2014. "Perinatally Acquired HIV Infection in Adolescents from Sub-Saharan Africa: A Review of Emerging Challenges." *The Lancet Infectious Diseases* 14 (7): 627–39. https://doi.org/10.1016/S1473-3099(13)70363-3.

Lowenthal, Elizabeth D, Haruna B Jibril, Mmapula L Sechele, Keofentse Mathuba, Ontibile Tshume, and Gabriel M Anabwani. 2014. "Disclosure of HIV Status to HIV-Infected Children in a Large African Treatment Center: Lessons Learned in Botswana." *Children and Youth Services Review*, Children and Youth Growing Up with HIV Infection in Sub-Saharan Africa: Implications for Health Service Delivery, 45 (October): 143–49. https://doi.org/10.1016/j.childyouth.2014.03.031.

Mandell, Nancy. 1988. "The Least-Adult Role in Studying Children." *Journal of Contemporary Ethnography* 16 (4): 433–67. https://doi.org/10.1177/0891241688164002.

Mehta, Supriya, Richard D. Moore, and Neil MH Graham. 1997. "Potential Factors Affecting Adherence with HIV Therapy." *Aids* 11 (14): 1665–1670.

Midtbø, Vivian, Violeth Shirima, Morten Skovdal, and Marguerite Daniel. 2012a. "How Disclosure and Antiretroviral Therapy Help HIV-Infected Adolescents in Sub-Saharan Africa Cope with Stigma." *African Journal of AIDS Research* 11 (3): 261–71. https://doi.org/10.2989/16085906.2012.734987.

———. 2012b. "How Disclosure and Antiretroviral Therapy Help HIV-Infected Adolescents in Sub-Saharan Africa Cope with Stigma." *African Journal of AIDS Research* 11 (3): 261–71. https://doi.org/10.2989/16085906.2012.734987.

Mkandawire-Valhmu, Lucy, Claire Wendland, Patricia E. Stevens, Peninnah M. Kako, Anne Dressel, and Jennifer Kibicho. 2013. "Marriage as a Risk Factor for HIV: Learning from the Experiences of HIV-Infected Women in Malawi." *Global Public Health* 8 (2): 187–201. https://doi.org/10.1080/17441692.2012.761261.

Murphy, Debra A., Kathleen J. Roberts, and Dannie Hoffman. 2002. "Stigma and Ostracism Associated with HIV/AIDS: Children Carrying the Secret of Their Mothers' HIV+ Serostatus." *Journal of Child and Family Studies* 11 (2): 191–202. https://doi.org/10.1023/A:1015177609382.

Ostrom, R. A., J. M. Serovich, J. Y. Lim, and T. L. Mason. 2006. "The Role of Stigma in Reasons for HIV Disclosure and Non-Disclosure to Children." *AIDS Care* 18 (1): 60–5. https://doi.org/10.1080/09540120500161769.

Parkhurst, Justin O. 2005. "The Response to HIV/AIDS and the Construction of National Legitimacy: Lessons from Uganda." *Development and Change* 36 (3): 571–90. https://doi.org/10.1111/j.0012-155X.2005.00424.x.

Pinzón-Iregui, María C., Consuelo M. Beck-Sagué, and Robert M. Malow. 2013. "Disclosure of Their HIV Status to Infected Children: A Review of the Literature." *Journal of Tropical Pediatrics* 59 (2): 84–89. https://doi.org/10.1093/tropej/fms052.

Rintamaki, Lance S., Terry C. Davis, Silvia Skripkauskas, Charles L. Bennett, and Michael S. Wolf. 2006. "Social Stigma Concerns and HIV Medication Adherence." *AIDS Patient Care & STDs* 20 (5): 359–368.

Schenk, Katie D., Karusa Kiragu, Julie Murugi, and Avina Sarna. 2014. "If You Build It, Will They Come? A Qualitative Investigation into Community Barriers to Accessing Paediatric HIV Services in Kenya." *Children and Youth Services Review*, Children and Youth Growing Up with HIV Infection in Sub-Saharan Africa: Implications for Health Service Delivery, 45 (October): 18–27. https://doi.org/10.1016/j.childyouth.2014.03.034.

Szelag, Barbara. 2011. "Growing Up with HIV: Disease Management among Perinatally Infected Adolescents." Doctoral Dissertation (Anthropology), Tampa, FL: University of Southern Florida. http://works.bepress.com/barbara_szelag/1/.

Tolan, Jenny. 2005. "Married Women and AIDS Vulnerability: Voices from Rural South Africa." *Stanford Undergraduate Research Journal*, Contemporary African Studies, Spring: 92–100.

Uganda AIDS Commission. 2014. "HIV and AIDS Uganda Country Progress Report - 2013." Kampala, Uganda: Uganda AIDS Commission. http://www.unaids.org/sites/default/files/country/documents//file%2C94771%2Cru..pdf.

———. 2015. "HIV and AIDS Uganda Country Progress Report - 2014." Kampala, Uganda: Uganda AIDS Commission. http://www.unaids.org/sites/default/files/country/documents/UGA_narrative_report_2015.pdf.

UNAIDS. 2015. "AIDSinfo." 2015. http://aidsinfo.unaids.org/.

Van Dyk, Alta C. 2010. "Treatment Adherence Following National Antiretroviral Rollout in South Africa." *African Journal of AIDS Research* 9 (3): 235–47. https://doi.org/10.2989/16085906.2010.530177.

Vreeman, Rachel C, Anna Maria Gramelspacher, Peter O Gisore, Michael L Scanlon, and Winstone M Nyandiko. 2013. "Disclosure of HIV Status to Children in Resource-Limited Settings: A Systematic Review." *Journal of the International AIDS Society* 16 (1). https://doi.org/10.7448/IAS.16.1.18466.

Walsh Lang, Colleen. 2019. "Flattening Need and Steepening Responsibility: Navigating Access to Islands of Care for Children Living with HIV in Uganda." In *Disadvantaged Childhoods and Humanitarian Intervention: Processes of Affective Commodification and Objectification*, edited by Kristen Cheney and Aviva Sinervo, 181–204. Palgrave Studies on Children and Development. Cham: Springer International Publishing. https://doi.org/10.1007/978-3-030-01623-4_8.

———. 2020. "Vulnerable Agents: Ugandan Children's Experiences with HIV Rehabilitation and Reintegration." *Arts & Sciences Electronic Theses and Dissertations*, May. https://doi.org/10.7936/cnvg-4796.

Whyte, Susan Reynolds, ed. 2014. *Second Chances: Surviving AIDS in Uganda*. Durham, NC: Duke University Press.

Chapter 4

Coordination of Medical Pluralism in Public HIV Health Care in South Africa

Shifting to an Alliance Framework with Traditional Health Practitioners

Claudia E. Ordóñez

Notwithstanding the political commitment to public health sector reform in South Africa brought by the end of apartheid, enduring developmental inequalities and inequities resulting from the colonial and apartheid systems have had a direct impact on the country's current burden of disease. At present, South Africa faces "a quadruple burden of disease including a dual [Human Immunodeficiency Virus (HIV) and tuberculosis] epidemic (about 17% of global burden), high maternal and child mortality (about 1% of global burden), high levels of violence and injuries (about 1.3% of global burden), and increasing noncommunicable diseases (about 1% of global burden)" (Malakoane et al. 2020, 2). Recent reviews and appraisals of the public health system in South Africa have diagnosed critical system vulnerabilities such as its aging and frail infrastructure and high shortage of staff and resources (Maphumulo and Bhengu 2019) and identified "negative staff attitudes, long waiting times, unclean facilities, medicine stock-outs, insufficient infection control and compromised safety and security of both staff and patients" as major challenges in the public health care sector (Malakoane et al. 2020, 2).

The burden of the HIV epidemic on South Africa as a whole has been immense. The country has the largest number of people with HIV (PWH) in the world, with 28.5% of all deaths attributable to AIDS in 2017 (Gona et al. 2020). It ranks third in the world for the highest HIV prevalence rate (20.4%, 2018 data) for adults aged 15–49 (UNAIDS 2020), with the epidemic disproportionately affecting certain population groups due to structural and contextual inequalities. These disparities can be seen in the differences in HIV prevalence between the different ethnic/population groups (0+ years of age) in South Africa: Black (16.6%), colored (5.3%), White (1.1%), and Indian/Asian (0.8%) (HSRC 2018). Presently, South African PWH are not dying at the high rate at which they were before the large-scale introduction of HIV antiretroviral drugs in 2004 and the implementation of universal prevention, testing, and treatment polices (Hansoti et al. 2019, 15). However, this public health achievement has resulted in an increasingly large number of HIV patients being funneled into a public health care system that struggles to link and retain them in treatment (Maphumulo and Bhengu 2019).

Another important contextual characteristic of health care in postcolonial and postapartheid South Africa is the existence of a *plural medical system*, by-product of the colonial and apartheid eras and often ignored, when not invalidated, by the Western hegemonic biomedical system. The concept of a plural medical system originated in Kleinman's 1978 explanatory model of medical systems as cultural systems and developed in medical anthropology as *medical pluralism* (Appelbaum Belisle et al. 2015, 3). Plural medical systems are often composed of biomedicine and other nonhegemonic medicines or healing practices, which are generally referred to as alternative, complementary, or traditional medicines, and used for health and illness.

The World Health Organization (WHO) defines traditional medicine as "the sum total of the knowledge, skills, and practices based on the theories, beliefs, and experiences indigenous to different cultures, whether explicable or not, used in the maintenance of health as well as in the prevention, diagnosis, improvement or treatment of physical and mental illness" (WHO 2013, 15). Traditional African medicine (TAM) is generally defined as "African or local medicine [that] has maintained certain core beliefs over time" (Flint 2008, 6).

TAM is a medical philosophy that understands disease as a "supernatural phenomenon governed by the hierarchy of vital powers beginning with a most powerful deity followed by lesser spiritual entities, ancestral spirits, living persons, animals, plants, and other objects. . . . Disharmony in these vital powers can cause illness" (Kale 1995, 1182). There are three different groups of practice in South African TAM defined by the mode of healing: *isangoma* (diviner), *inyanga* (herbalist), and *umthandazi* (prophet or faith healer) (Appelbaum Belisle et al. 2015, 4). According to Kale (1995, 1182), *isangomas* are diviners who determine the cause of illness by using ancestral spirits, and most of them are female. Isangomas cannot choose to become diviners; they have to be called by the ancestors to become one. A chosen individual behaves like a person with mental illness during the calling period, and only a skilled diviner can differentiate this behavior. Their training can take between a few weeks to up to 10 years, depending on the ability of the apprentice, and includes having skills similar to those of an inyanga or herbalist. *Inyangas*, who are mostly males, possess extensive knowledge about curative herbs and medicine of animal origin. An inyanga chooses to become one. Finally, *umthandazis* are professed Christians employing faith as a means of healing. They belong to one of the independent African churches and heal by prayer, using holy water or ash, or by touching the patient (Kale 1995, 1182). PWH in South Africa seek the services of all, some, or only one of these different types of THPs depending on their personal preferences and body, mind, and spiritual needs (Appelbaum Belisle et al. 2015).

This chapter describes the relationship between biomedicine and TAM in the treatment and care of HIV in South Africa and suggests harnessing medical pluralism through alliance and coordination between TAM and biomedicine. Based on my own research and experience,[1] I propose that one important barrier to sustainably manage the antiretroviral therapy (ART) program in South Africa is the insufficient recognition and acceptance of the strong plurality characterizing the health-seeking behaviors of HIV patients. The argument developed here offers a rationale for why a model of HIV care that is culturally and contextually appropriate and that channels the benefits resulting from an *alliance* between TAM and biomedicine deserves serious consideration.

The integration of individual interests in the context of South Africa's medical plurality seems to have proven an impossibility when dealing with the often divergent interests of the two very different cosmologies[2] in which TAM and biomedicine are embedded, namely traditional African and Western (Hammond-Tooke 1989). Largely unsuccessful partnerships attempting to unilaterally integrate or merge TAM into biomedicine have been the most commonly used strategy in South African public HIV health care since the beginning of the epidemic in the early 1980s. In contrast, conceptualizing the relationship between TAM and biomedicine as a power-sharing alliance provides a framework for a collaboration between both healing practices that could bring mutual gain and the achievement of the common goal of health and well-being for the patient. A power-sharing alliance framework would preserve their independent interests and respect their different cosmologies.

Further, and borrowing from the psychoanalytic conceptualization of "working alliance" (Bordin 1979), an alliance framework to harness South Africa's medical pluralism could include features such as agreement on goals, assignment of tasks, and development of bonds between the two medicines, as well as incorporate the concept of *ally* from social justice theory to model the role of biomedicine in the state of being allied with TAM. The suggested alliance framework emphasizes power sharing and complementarity instead of merging (partnership) or integrating approaches. Implementing the alliance framework to synergize the capabilities of TAM and biomedicine in advancing their common goal of health and well-being for PWH could also have positive implications beyond HIV care in South Africa.

The perspective presented here is the product of professional and personal experiences in South Africa beginning in 2004. Since 2009, I have been involved as a researcher in collaborative anthropological and biomedical research on the sociocultural aspects of HIV treatment in the province of KwaZulu-Natal among PWH who self-identify as of Zulu ethnicity. These research collaborations have largely focused on identifying risk factors for virologic failure[3] to ART and have been carried out through case-control studies employing epidemiological, quantitative, and qualitative methods (including participant observation, different interviewing techniques, and grounded theory). The collaborations have also included public health ethnographic research among Zulu PWH, Zulu TAM practitioners (or traditional health practitioners [THPs]), and a variety of biomedical HIV health care providers.

The analysis of the South African plural health system in this chapter will be limited to the binary of TAM and biomedicine, since the relationship between these two constitutes the thrust of the research we have conducted during the past decade in the KwaZulu-Natal province. It is important to mention that other nonhegemonic medicines and health practices coexist with TAM within the South African plural health system (e.g., Hindu, Ayurvedic, and Islamic medical practices), and that the binary of biomedicine and TAM is not intended to ratify the false dualism between modernity and traditionalism. Furthermore, the term "traditional" is used with the understanding that it does not imply timelessness, rigidity, and/or a static state. Most people of African descent in South Africa use traditional to acknowledge aspects of local African culture maintained over time.

Finally, this chapter will use the definition articulated by Benton, Sangaramoorthy, and Kalofonos (2017) for the category of "postcolonial," where this term not only refers to a time, location, group of people, or intergroup relations but also signals how "notions of the objective, the authoritative, and the universal have been shaped by a history of (Western) technoscientific interventions that have influenced assumptions about difference, modernity, and the future" (Benton, Sangaramoorthy, and Kalofonos 2017, 3).

In order to provide context for the argument of channeling medical pluralism in South Africa toward confluence and alliance between THPs and biomedical practitioners, I will start by briefly describing the importance of South African history in understanding the current HIV health care context in the country. This section will be followed by a summary of global HIV health care narratives that have informed and shaped biomedical discourses and responses to the HIV epidemic in contemporary South Africa. To situate medical pluralism in the context of responses to HIV treatment in postcolonial South Africa, the chapter will also describe the "postcolonial paradox" and the challenges and importance of balancing power between TAM and biomedicine in HIV health care provision. Following the description of TAM in HIV care in South Africa, there will be a description of the need for effectively implementing a context responsive "people-centered" approach to health care and the role of TAM and its practitioners on community-level responses to HIV treatment in South Africa. The last two sections of the chapter will explore the advantages of fostering a power-sharing alliance framework between TAM and biomedicine as well as implementing plurality coordination through government policies to support the alliance model between the two medicines.

SOUTH AFRICAN HISTORY, TAM, AND HIV

Understanding the ripple effects of South African history in the present day is crucial for contextualizing the HIV epidemic. Historical events and processes triggered with the arrival of European colonizers to South Africa have impacted structural conditions and the cultures of native populations, including indigenous practices related to health, sickness, and healing. Consideration and awareness of these events are crucial for understanding and contextualizing medical pluralism in South Africa, as well as for supporting the argument for plural coordination and shifting toward an alliance between TAM and biomedicine.

European colonial ruling in South Africa began with the Dutch in 1652 and continued by the British starting in 1795. Its mutation into the apartheid regime formally established around the mid-1900s "led to lasting and deepening poverty, inequality and underfunded medical systems, among other crucial factors associated with the [HIV] epidemic. Black, Indian and Coloured communities were separated (between and within) and isolated from each other and white populations; in this process of relocation, individuals and whole communities lost their land, other property, and familial and social groups" (Ordóñez and Marconi 2012, 3–4). Among these three communities, Black South Africans ended up with the greatest burden of injustice. Almost 30 years after the end of apartheid, the democratization of South Africa, and the election of a largely Black government, the ripples of colonialism continue to have an impact on Black South Africans, who, despite having always been the majority population in the country, still experience greater inequality in securing basic human rights such as adequate education, shelter, and health (Statistics South Africa, 2011; Baker 2019; International Monetary Fund, 2020).

Among the many power struggles between indigenous black South Africans and Europeans, the provision of health care has been a contested area since the early days of the colonial rule (Flint 2008). Historical accounts reveal that TAM practices have been documented as part of indigenous South African cultures since the time of early contacts with Western Europeans, and they have long been a source of contention between Western medical practitioners and THPs as well as a target of criminal actions by European colonial rulers (Pimenova 2019; Flint 2008). Despite the oppressive forces and criminalizing tactics of the political system, ethnohistorical research indicates the continuous relevance of TAM in health-seeking behaviors among precolonial indigenous groups in South Africa (Flint 2008). THPs often constitute the first contact patients have with health care, past and present (Appelbaum Belisle et al. 2015).

The centuries long, continuous relevance of TAM among black South Africans demonstrates its depth and strength as a cultural healing practice for body and mind. TAM has also been used as an adaptive strategy to survive and counter colonizing dominant narratives and hegemonic systems. The contextual relevance and importance of TAM is essential to understanding the emergence of the HIV epidemic in South Africa. This epidemic imposed an overwhelming burden on the public health care sector, while situating THPs front and center because of their relevance and strategic positioning for health promotion and HIV prevention, given their large numbers and geographical distribution. Often, THPs were (and are) the only health care providers available in many of the remote rural areas of the country.

Scholars have attributed South Africa's large proportion of individuals living with HIV to historical processes and contextual factors converging with the emergence of the HIV epidemic around 1982 (Hodes 2018; Abdool Karim and Abdool Karim 2002). Political factors such as heightened repression and resulting discriminatory laws during the end of apartheid in the 1980s and HIV denialism during the 1990s and early 2000s are often identified in the literature as culprits of the epidemic by having delayed the national response to the emergence of HIV (Cichocki 2020; Ordóñez and Marconi 2012). Other factors have also been important in the spread of HIV in this region (Abdool Karim and Abdool Karim 2002; Fassin and Schneider 2003). "Extensive research has examined the influence of individual movement due to migratory labor, the commercial sex trade along major highway trucking routes, gender violence/inequality, and the prevalence of multiple concurrent partnerships" (Ordóñez and Marconi 2012, 4). Additionally, HIV-related stigma has become a barrier for individuals to disclose their status to their partners or seek care and treatment (Ordóñez and Marconi 2012, 4). Black indigenous people in South Africa have found themselves in a vulnerable position as a result of the structural violence inflicted through Western dominance, exploitation, and segregation starting nearly 400 years ago and augmented by recent historical events, such as the emergence of HIV, the political upheaval during the end of the apartheid era, and the subsequent HIV denialism.

The dual use of TAM and biomedicine by patients with HIV in South Africa since the early stages of the epidemic during the 1990s is confirmed by scholarly publications from the health and social sciences (Appelbaum Belisle et al. 2015; Mokgobi 2013). Bringing biomedical and traditional health care together for PWH in the early 1990s was also supported in Africa by the WHO, when during this time the organization "recommended that traditional medicine be included in national responses to HIV" (UNAIDS 2007). "Early attempts to combine the best of both systems included a variety of projects [including some in South Africa] that looked at the usefulness of traditional herbal remedies for the treatment of HIV-related illnesses. Studies looking at traditional healers' perceptions of sexually transmitted infections and HIV infection were also conducted. With this information, collaborative projects began, training traditional healers as educators and counsellors to disseminate information on HIV and sexually transmitted infections in their communities and to their peers" (UNAIDS 2007).

The use of two medicines for HIV purposes has continued into the twenty first century. In its efforts to reverse the HIV epidemic, the South African Department of Health has been recognizing the role of THPs as a key resource in HIV health care, alongside biomedical and behavioral interventions (Zuma et al. 2018). Given their positionality as community members who share the same cultural identity of their patients as well as their physical location in communities, THPs have proven to be very effective in addressing and managing issues related to stigma that often prevent people from getting tested and accessing care, with about 80% of Black indigenous South Africans seeking healing from the TAM system (Zuma et al. 2018). TAM is also used by PWH for reasons unrelated to HIV, and studies have identified its critical role for psychosocial and spiritual counseling and communicating with ancestors (Appelbaum Belisle et al. 2015).

In 2007, the South African government approved the *South African Traditional Health Practitioners Act* (THP Act of 2007). This Act defined "traditional health practice as performance of a function, activity, process, or service based on a traditional philosophy that uses indigenous African techniques and principles that include traditional medicine or practice, including the physical or mental preparation of an individual for puberty, adulthood, pregnancy, childbirth, and death" (Peltzer 2009, 956). More specifically, the Act was aimed:

- to establish the Interim Traditional Health Practitioners Council of South Africa;

- to provide for a regulatory framework to ensure the efficacy, safety, and quality of traditional health care services;
- to provide for the management and control over the registration, training, and conduct of practitioners, students, and specified categories in the THP profession. (South African Government 2007)

The THP Act of 2007 allows the registration of four categories of THPs: herbalist (*inyanga* or *amaxhwele*), diviner (*isangoma* or *amagqirha*), traditional surgeons (*iingcibi*) who mainly do circumcisions, and traditional birth attendants (*ababelethisi* or *abazalisi*). The spiritual or faith healer (*umthandazi*) category was not included in the Act (Peltzer 2009).

South Africa has made progress toward the inclusion of TAM into the national health care system by the enactment of the THP Act of 2007 and measures such as "a traditional medicine directorate within the Department of Health, a traditional medicine research institute, postgraduate education in herbal science, and a draft policy for the institutionalisation of African traditional medicine, including a national institute" (Peltzer 2009, 957). However, serious issues in the operationalization of the THP Act and a lack of a government-supported strategic plan for the conceptualization of the relationship between TAM and biomedicine are some of the powerful factors that continue to perpetuate the rift between the two medicines, which currently operate separately and in parallel within the general context of South African health care, as well as in the specific area of HIV care. Meanwhile, Black indigenous South Africans continue to use TAM and biomedicine for HIV purposes while having to navigate and negotiate on their own the unaddressed and persistent power struggle between THPs and biomedical providers.

THE IMPACTS OF THE SOUTH AFRICAN HEALTH CARE SYSTEM AND GLOBAL HEALTH HIV NARRATIVES

Country-specific structural inequalities and inequities impact many national health systems around the world. The HIV epidemic in South Africa offers a clear and devastating example of how systemic oppression and racism produce vulnerable populations, which are often the most affected by any type of natural or social crisis. The persistence of structural inequalities since colonial times is a key factor in the origin and maintenance of the HIV epidemic among Black South Africans, especially Black females, who experience the added burden of gender power dynamics (Mabaso et al. 2019).

Around the year 2010 global health organizations dedicated to the HIV epidemic started promoting the narrative of the "end of AIDS" (Sangaramoorthy

2018). In 2012, the XIX International AIDS Conference adopted the slogan "Turning the Tide Together," signifying that a concerted effort had begun to end the epidemic. However, these announcements and objectives were critiqued by some HIV researchers at that time, who noted that despite the progress made in curbing the epidemic it was "important to highlight that within certain communities [incidence] rates actually increased" (Ordóñez and Marconi 2012, 1). A 2011 UNAIDS report on the last 30 years of the epidemic also warned about the "the considerable variation in HIV prevalence and epidemiological patterns within countries," pointing to the existence of "epidemic hotspots" (Ordóñez and Marconi 2012, 1). More recently, some researchers in the field of HIV are also using the concept of "HIV microepidemics" to describe the spatially and socially circumscribed nature of epidemic hotspots (Krebs et al. 2019). "Hotspots exist among men who have sex with men (MSM), ethnic minorities, young women, injection drug users (IDUs) and population groups historically subject to significant inequality" (Ordóñez and Marconi 2012, 1).

Both global health homogenizing narratives (*End of AIDS*) and local narratives (*HIV microepidemics*) can be problematic. While global narratives are the by-product of the hegemonic global health system exercising authority and control over human existence to the detriment of autonomy and diversity, local narratives that acknowledge the importance and necessity of micro-contextualization can have the unintended effect of otherizing people and communities by imposing labels and conceptualizations that can result in stigmatizing groups within societies. For example, using the conceptualization of hotspots can be useful to identify and understand local epidemiological phenomena, but simultaneously run the risk of creating discriminatory labels by imposing ideas of radical difference or otherness on communities experiencing high rates of HIV, with the public global health imagination implicitly stigmatizing difference through a common characterization (Benton, Sangaramoorthy, and Kalofonos 2017). The conceptualization of hotspots and HIV microepidemics implicitly (and sometimes explicitly) uses elements of sociocultural identity, unintendedly justifying and promoting ideas of otherness.

While buzz terms and conceptualizations incorporate the concern for the disproportionate burdens experienced by certain groups in society, the global and public health fields have not paid enough attention to the tension between distinct sociohistorical contexts and ethnocentric bias. This tension has a significant impact on HIV prevention and treatment among certain groups of people. Perceptions of radical difference have influenced global and public health responses and are linked to a tacit otherness in the biased Western conceptualization of groups of people who are disproportionally affected by HIV and AIDS, resulting in unintended consequences for the recipients of HIV programs.

International development and global health systems recently transitioned from the era of the Millennium Development Goals (MDGs), which took place from 2000 to 2015, to the era of Sustainable Development Goals or "post-2015" era, which has the year 2030 as target for achievement of the goals (Yamey et al. 2016). The planning of the *post-2015* era has been carried out primarily by influential Western academicians, think tanks, and international development organizations and then adopted by the United Nations system. "Global Development Assistance for Health (DAH) increased substantially in the MDGs era, from US $10.8 billion in 2001 to $28.1 billion by 2012 (in 2010 US dollars), and it played a crucial role in tackling global challenges such as HIV/AIDS and malaria" (Yamey et al. 2016, 125). The impact of increasing global development assistance for health can be seen in the development of South Africa's sizable ART program.

South Africa has the "most high-profile HIV epidemic in the world, with an estimated 7.7 million people living with HIV in 2018" (Avert 2019, n.p.). Twenty years after international acknowledgment of an HIV epidemic taking place in the country, the introduction of government-subsidized ART for South African PWH in 2004 resulted in a significant positive change in the dynamics of the epidemic. These changes have lowered the rate of mother-to-child transmission and increased the national life expectancy by six years.

With over four million HIV patients, South Africa currently has the largest national public sector ART program in the world (Avert 2020; Meyer-Rath et al. 2017). The United States' "President's Emergency Plan for AIDS Relief" (PEPFAR), which underwrote the South African ART program, has been considered "the most ambitious and successful global public health program since smallpox eradication" (Katz, Bassett, and Wright 2013, 1). After almost a decade of financial support and a successful implementation of the ART program, the US government announced in 2012 that "it would cut South Africa's PEPFAR budget in half by 2017, making South Africa the first PEPFAR-funded country to transition to full ownership of—and financial responsibility for—its HIV program" (Katz, Bassett, and Wright 2013, 1).

Since this announcement, the South African government has been progressively financing the ART program with domestic resources, and in 2015 it was investing more than $1.34 billion annually to run its HIV programs (South African Government 2018). At the same time, the government has been closing many of the specialized HIV treatment health facilities created by PEPFAR, "moving patients into government-run, community-based health care centers, where long waiting times and medication shortages are common" (Katz, Bassett, and Wright 2013, 1). Changing the nature of the South African ART program from an emergency response financed by foreign aid to an "independent," South African-financed response has meant adopting a neoliberal health care system model for integration of services largely designed by few and selected stakeholders based on high-income (World Bank Index), Western countries (e.g., the 2013 "Lancet Commission on Investing in Health").

Similarly, global public health campaigns introduced in South Africa don't prioritize or appropriately acknowledge local cultural and social contexts. In the setting of South Africa's public ART program, "notions of progress that separate West from Rest" (Benton, Sangaramoorthy, and Kalofonos 2017) prevail in the relationship between biomedical and public health providers and PWH, who are overwhelmingly poor Black South Africans. Benton, Sangaramoorthy, and Kalofonos define logics of "Project Time" and "Adherence Time," as expressions of the linkage between power, temporality, and the Positive Living global health narrative in the context of HIV programs and interventions (2017). A booklet developed by Johns Hopkins University for health communications in Africa describes Positive Living as "taking care of your health and body when you have HIV. A person with HIV can live a healthy, normal, and productive life when they practice Positive Living" (2013).

The South African ART program, carried out within the public health care system, exemplifies these logics by constantly experiencing and circulating ideas of scarcity, uncertainty, fear of failure, and crisis. A quote from an ART stakeholder also exemplifies the logics of project time and adherence time when listing what the idea of "Positive Living" promotes:

> Coming out and declaring your status publicly to help others overcome stigma and promote that you can live normally with HIV when on ART—to increase the numbers of VL [viral load] tests done, patients have been given a VL anniversary date to empower them to demand that the test be done. (ART program key stakeholder, personal communication, November 2019)

Similar to strategies employed by other ART programs using the Positive Living narrative, South African PWH are constantly reminded of the critical importance of synchronizing their lives to the logics of project and adherence and of fully assuming responsibility for themselves: being both subjects and agents, dependent and self-sufficient. *Positive Living* becomes thus a "highly expressive negotiation of a neoliberal ethos of self-sufficiency under receding or crumbling state social services" (Benton, Sangaramoorthy, and Kalofonos 2017, 10).

Another important aspect of the Positive Living narrative exemplified in the quote above ("Coming out and declaring your status publicly") is the promotion of confessional technologies and therapeutic citizenship (access to networks and their resources), which are cornerstone strategies used by HIV activists and biomedical health workers and development organizations implementing HIV and AIDS interventions (Nichaus 2018). With deep European social and historical roots, confessional technologies are also connected to coming out narratives that emerged among LGBTQ+ communities in the United States during the 1960s promoting the idea of acceptance and liberation through words (Nichaus 2018, 67). "In the context of HIV/AIDS, confessional technologies comprise voluntary counseling and testing (VCT), 'coming out' with HIV positivity, and providing public testimony about sickness and the positive transformative effects of medication" (Nichaus 2018, 67).

The use of the confessional technologies strategy in rural areas of South Africa can be culturally inappropriate and ineffective due to differences between social and cosmological contexts. Anthropologist Isak Nichaus warns against "the assumption that confessional technologies—such as coming out with an HIV+ identity—provide a universally appropriate means of confronting the AIDS epidemic" (Nichaus 2018, 85). In his book *AIDS in the Shadow of Biomedicine*, Nichaus provides a powerful quote from a male participant in his ethnographic research in rural South Africa between the years 2003 and 2004:

> I hate to be tested. I hate to know that I'm going to die. I hate people telling me that I am HIV-positive. It will be a problem because I will worry too much. When the disease and the worries get together, I will be mourning too much. I will be fighting two battles. (Nichaus 2018, 67)

The testimony of this male from rural South Africa exemplifies what researchers have described as the "silence, secrecy and coded talk as responses to HIV/AIDS in various parts of South Africa's rural periphery" (Nichaus 2018, 68). Data from our HIV ethnographic research in the South African province of KwaZulu-Natal have shown similar reactions from PWH living in rural areas. Between 2018 and 2019 our team conducted a research project in peri-urban and rural KwaZulu-Natal in collaboration with a local program called Integration of TB in Education and Care for HIV/AIDS and entitled "Barriers to HIV Viral Load Monitoring in KwaZulu-Natal and the Impact of Traditional Health Practitioners." An excerpt from one of our interviews with nurses working in the public health sector exemplifies similar attitudes toward denial, defiance, and the choice of remaining ignorant about one's HIV status:

INTERVIEWER: What made someone feel uncomfortable going to the clinic? Has a patient ever told you something like that?

NURSE: And, em, last year, the experience I had, this was the first time though, it wasn't of those, em, Makhosis,[4] it was the religion. This lady came because she

> was forced by her husband to come and test. . . . Anyway, the husband tested at work and found out that he's positive. But he didn't tell, expose, disclose the status to wife, and wife was sick. He brought the wife and said, "go to the clinic and test for HIV." She came, and tested. She was also positive, but her belief was very strong. Their religion belief was very strong than anything else. She didn't believe in those results or anything. The first thing she said when she got these results was, she wasn't angry or anything at husband, she said, "I'm going to pray, my God will change these results to negative." She said she doesn't believe in tablets. Husband, he has been forcing her, so she is not prepared to take any medication, she's going to pray. And she wanted to test again because she has been praying all these months. She wants to know if, eh, the results have been changed now to negative. Anyway, we said "Okay, it's fine, we're going to test you again." We tested her; it was still positive. And she said, "No, that means I didn't pray, eh, well. I still need to pray more and, em, to my God because I know that my God is going to change these results to negative. So that's the issue." (April 2019, KwaZulu-Natal. Project's data analysis in progress, field investigator and interviewer: Diana Jeang)

Although Nichaus's research participant gave his statement in the context of a pre-ART national program time, when lifesaving HIV medications were scarce everywhere and mostly available through out-of-pocket purchase, its validity still holds today, as can be seen in the above excerpt. Due to irregular stockpiling in government health centers and the limited number and coverage of health care facilities, availability of ART has often been scarce in rural areas after the launch of the 2004 government-subsidized ART program for South African PWH. In the rural context, governmental policies and their implementation are generally what secures access to therapeutic resources rather than employing confessional behaviors. Global health homogenizing narratives often ignore these important differences in local contexts and populations, consequentially affecting the efficacy of HIV prevention, care, and treatment interventions.

THE "POSTCOLONIAL PARADOX" AND THE TRADITIONAL AFRICAN MEDICAL SYSTEM

In her book *Ancestors and Antiretrovirals: The Biopolitics of HIV/AIDS in Post-Apartheid South Africa*, Clair Decoteau (2013) describes the "postcolonial paradox" in South Africa and its relevance to the HIV epidemic: "The dilemma that all postcolonial states face of attempting to sustain a national identity in the face of the deterritorializing forces of globalization is heightened in South Africa for several reasons: its late transition from colonialism, its efforts to maintain its position as an economic leader on the African continent, and its need to deal successfully with the mutual pandemics of AIDS and poverty" (7).

The idea of postcolonial paradox explains South Africa's contradictory reality of acquiescing to demands of the neoliberal era to compete in the world market while simultaneously attempting to address inequity and inequality and promote a pan-Africanist renaissance. The influence of this paradox can be recognized in the South African health care system, an exclusively biomedical health care system that in theory acknowledges and accepts traditional African approaches (e.g., THP Act of 2007) to health care.

Oseni and Shannon conducted a systematic qualitative review to explore the relationship between indigenous health practitioners (IHPs) and allopathic (or biomedical) health practitioners (AHPs) in Africa and to elucidate implications of the nature of the relationship for future collaboration (2020). This review of the literature found that the relationship between IHPs and AHPs in the plural medical context of Africa is defined by a power struggle that originated in the power differential brought by European colonization (Oseni and Shannon 2020). This power struggle is a hindrance to the collaboration between indigenous and biomedical practitioners "and as such could partly account for the limited success of efforts to foster collaboration to date" (Oseni and Shannon 2020, 1).

While the South African public health system acknowledges both biomedical and TAM approaches to HIV care, it only consistently supports the biomedical model of care. The lack of a decisive governmental strategy for implementing the THP Act of 2007 demonstrates how the power struggles identified by Oseni and Shannon (2020) have not been addressed. The implementation of this Act has not only been slow but also avoided clearly defining who is a THP and providing a thorough and well-organized plan to implement accreditation of THPs in the country. This situation perpetuates the power differential between THPs and biomedical practitioners and continues to promote the long-tested (and mostly failed) strategy of integrating THPs to lower subordinate positions of biomedical health care provision. The integration strategy has consisted in training THPs in biomedical understandings of HIV and AIDS to provide community-based HIV care, promotion and distribution of condoms, and coordination of ART adherence (Zuma et al. 2018).

In the entanglement of postcolonial paradoxes, the historical power differentials between medicines become perpetuated by accepting the validity of both the biomedical and traditional approaches to health and healing without addressing the hegemony and hierarchy of biomedicine. Attempts to create an accreditation system following the enactment of the THP Act have failed and TAM is still unregulated because of the lack of accreditation procedures. Additionally, there has been a lack of effort to allow for cross referral and joint care: "Although the Department [of Health] supports a system of collaboration on Primary Health Care and HIV and AIDS prevention and education, at present the Department does not support referrals from the formal health system to traditional healers, principally because of a lack of research and regulation around the dosage and efficacy of traditional treatments" (Peltzer 2009, 957). This situation translates into an added burden to PWH navigating the public health care system, with the battle to resolve the paradoxes of postcolonialism "waged on the terrain of AIDS politics" (Decoteau 2013, 7).

For almost 20 years, there has been a struggle between the national health care system, global health and international development stakeholders, and indigenous healers over the signification of HIV and AIDS in the South African context. The metaphorical use of *modernity* and *traditionalism* has been rearticulated in the postapartheid era to organize power within the context of the HIV epidemic. The conceptualization of modernity and traditionalism also informs what Decoteau (2013) calls the *myth of incommensurability*, "the ideology that indigenous (read 'traditional') and biomedical (read 'modern') forms of healing are irreconcilably incompatible" (Decoteau 2013, 8). In the context of South Africa's plural health system, the tension between modernity and traditionalism and the resulting myth of incommensurability represent another incarnation of the paradoxes of postcolonialism.

The myth of incommensurability is mostly embraced by biomedical practitioners and nonindigenous segments of the South African population. In contrast, the tension between modernity and traditionalism is not an issue for THPs and Black indigenous South Africans; it is rather understood as an opportunity or asset. A biomedical and anthropological research collaboration looking at TAM use among ART patients in the city of Durban, KwaZulu-Natal, documented patients' concurrent use of the biomedical and TAM systems and concluded that "among patients, there was a nuanced understanding of TAM's utility in the context of their management of HIV. Specifically, patients and providers in this study illustrated that TAM does not necessarily undermine adherence to ART and further, that TAM is not limited to herbal treatments that are ingested" (Appelbaum Belisle et al. 2015, 13–14). Findings in this study suggested that TAM had both concurrent and complementary roles for ART patients using both medicines and worked in tandem with biomedicine for different purposes: "To conflate the independent identities of TAM use for cultural reasons with TAM use for HIV management is to lose the nuanced distinctions that characterised TAM use for patients like those in this study population" (Appelbaum Belisle et al. 2015, 13).

The power struggle and the organization of power among the different modern and traditional actors of South Africa's plural health system surrounding the signification of HIV and AIDS are manifested through the establishment of hierarchical ranking and boundaries for the appropriate functions for each of the main actors participating in the provision of health care. Exerting its hegemonic positionality in the health care system, this ranking is determined and imposed by biomedicine. Most of the collaborations between TAM and biomedicine for purposes of HIV-related health care have been founded on the assumption that THPs will be brought into biomedicine to be trained, certified, and validated within the superior and safer biomedical and scientific paradigm (Oseni and Shannon 2020; Zuma et al. 2018). The assertion of the dominance of Western cosmology, whether explicit or implicit, is also demonstrated by feelings of superiority and prejudice frequently present among biomedical practitioners and manifested in perceptions of themselves in the roles of teacher, supervisor, or instructor to THPs when in the context of TAM and biomedical collaborations (Oseni and Shannon 2020, 6–7). Collaborations are usually designed for THPs to support HIV care and treatment, assuming the role of boots on the ground to implement community health biomedical interventions, limiting their role to health promotion activities: "In addition to healing of the mind, body and spirit, THPs serve many roles in the community, including counselling, social mediation, cultural education and being custodians of African traditions and customs" (Mothibe and Sibanda 2019, 7). The expression and assertion of power by practitioners of the biomedical system often takes the form of implicit or explicit paternalistic attitudes and narratives. This situation of marked power imbalance is accentuated by the ethnocentric approach to inquiry used among biomedical stakeholders interested in exploring and understanding the TAM system, who seek to evaluate (and potentially validate) the indigenous system by using the scientific paradigm, which is epistemologically problematic to understand and evaluate indigenous cosmologies.

PEOPLE-CENTERED HEALTH CARE

The book *When People Come First*, edited by Biehl and Petryna (2013), argues for a more comprehensive, people-centered approach to global health, bringing to the forefront the key approach of looking for solutions among communities themselves. The people-centered model has been adopted by WHO, which currently advocates for *people-centered health services* and defines these as "an approach to care that consciously adopts the perspectives of individuals, families and communities, and sees them as participants as well as beneficiaries of trusted health systems that respond to their needs and preferences in humane and holistic ways" (WHO 2019). From the perspective of the WHO, people-centered care is organized around the health needs and expectations of people (what matters to them) rather than organized around diseases, and it is seen as provided in partnership with people rather than given to people.

Although this more recent narrative from the global health system points in the right direction, there seems to be a gap between the theory of people-centered care and the reality of its implementation in global health and development interventions. These interventions tend to lack acknowledgment of power dynamics between benefactors and beneficiaries or among partners, resulting in unaddressed hierarchical relationships between different types of health care stakeholders that hinder the effectiveness of programs in member states of the WHO such as South Africa (Mothibe and Sibanda 2019). As discussed in the above section explaining the postcolonial paradox, the dominance exerted by the South African biomedical system, through both the unilateral conceptualization of an "integrative" model for health care collaboration and its prejudicial and hierarchical approach to relationships with THP stakeholders, serves as an example of the gap between theory and practice of the recommended people-centered approach to health services.

THPs in South Africa should be considered key stakeholders in the design and implementation of health care interventions that look for solutions among communities themselves. In many Black South African communities, people feel hesitant to use the government's local health clinics for HIV-related services due to common experiences of rude or unhelpful health care staff and of socioeconomic discrimination or stigma. Relatedly, research has shown the important role of community-level factors associated with HIV treatment. Social support networks, cultural and gender norms, and stigma and discrimination have been identified as the most important factors for the HIV treatment cascade (Moshabela et al. 2016). TAM and its practitioners are an example of support networks and cultural norms impacting the HIV treatment cascade in South Africa. A systematic qualitative review of the literature assessing collaborative efforts between THPs and the South African biomedical health care system in the context of the HIV health care found that "THPs are held in high esteem in local communities and deliver care to patients in a culturally familiar setting" (Pimenova 2019).

ALLIANCE (INSTEAD OF INTEGRATION) WITH THPS

Shifting the relationship with THPs from the partnership model to an alliance framework could be a more effective strategy to operationalize WHO's recommended people-centered approach to health care while supporting people's preference for medical pluralism. This shift would account for key factors driving people's health-seeking preferences and behaviors that would otherwise be missed. Mallett's research in Sierra Leone suggests that accounting for these factors is "as important for long-term efforts to prevent public health challenges like undernutrition as it is for attempts to contain outbreaks of deadly viruses such as Ebola" (Mallett 2014, para. 5). Mallet also points to the "power of relationships" characteristic of TAM: THPs "who have been operating for years and are deeply embedded within the social fabric of communities have often accumulated considerable trust among local people" (2014, para. 4). THPs in South Africa not only offer the power of an already trustful, culturally relevant relationship with the community, but they also live among the community, including communities located in remote rural areas with little or no access to health services given the historical shortages of biomedical providers and other resources in the South African public health care system.

The urgency and pressures brought by the start of the massive ART program in 2004 resulted, for the first time in recent history, in significant attention from national health care system stakeholders toward the country's THPs. THPs were approached with a utilitarian view, seen as quickly deployable health care system agents to help improve access to HIV treatment and support HIV education. This approach to collaboration for the advancement of the ART agenda, which has been since then mostly described as a partnership integrating THPs to the public health care system, has rarely been easy or sustainable. The model for coordination with THPs in the context of HIV care has been unilaterally conceived and is riddled with implicit and explicit ethnocentric bias that reflects the status quo of historical power differentials between the two medicines. This hegemonic integrative partnership model for plurality coordination has been shown to be ineffective both in South Africa and in many places of the African continent (Oseni and Shannon 2020). Approaching plurality coordination between two very different cosmologies with integrative or merging goals has turned into a missed opportunity for synergizing medical plurality in the South African context.

Well-described and documented in Karen Flint's book about African medicine in South Africa, TAM and biomedicine cultures have different approaches to the understanding of the body and the origin of illness while sharing a history of commercial and ideological competition and different relations to state power (2012, 183). This history of competition offers another element of justification for conceptualizing the collaboration between THPs and the biomedical system as an alliance instead of as a partnership. A relationship in which key independent interests are preserved and sharing power is approached as complementary, in contrast to a relationship that seeks to unilaterally integrate and merge, disregarding the individual interests of the weakest partner in the relationship. A complementary approach combines the distinct capabilities of TAM and biomedicine while acknowledging and respecting their different cosmologies to advance the common goal of health and well-being for PWH.

The psychoanalytic conceptualization of "working alliance" (Bordin 1979) offers a tested and apt approach to the design of an alliance framework. The working alliance includes features such as agreement on goals, assignment of tasks, and development of bonds. Additionally, also incorporating the concept of *ally* to model the role of biomedicine in a working alliance with TAM could have a transformative effect through the development of positive bonds between practitioners of the two medicines that could contribute to address unresolved power differentials. Allyship is characterized by an active, accountable, consistent, and long-term practice of unlearning and reevaluating current power structures and hierarchies with the understanding that the party in the position of privilege and power seeks to operate in solidarity with a marginalized group. An allyship in the context of the relationship between biomedical practitioners and THPs could provide an effective platform to understand, respect, and adapt to the perspectives of others who have traditionally been oppressed.

An allyship approach to collaborations between TAM and biomedicine in the context of medical pluralism and the HIV epidemic in South Africa could address the issue of incommensurability of indigenous and biomedical forms of knowledge and healing by avoiding comparisons and competition between partners, thus shifting the emphasis toward acknowledging and attempting to balance power dynamics in the relationship. By not focusing on comparisons, allyship also deemphasizes perceptions of difference and changes the narrative about tacit otherness in the conceptualization of groups of people.

MEDICAL PLURALITY COORDINATION

Shim (2017) did a comparative cross-national meta-analysis of the behavioral consequences of plural logics of action based on the empirical case of plural medical systems—defined as the binary of biomedicine and alternative medicine. This study found that "plural systems affect health outcomes negatively when tensions between biomedicine and alternative medicine are unaddressed. In contrast, plural systems produce tangible health benefits when biomedicine and alternative medicine are coordinated through government policies or by health care organizations/professionals" (Shim 2017, 1). Given that institutional settings influence the subjective user expectations and the objective health care outcomes, the health care outcomes of settings with plural medical systems depend on how the logics of the different medicines are managed by health care institutions or systems (Shim 2017, 16). Shim proposes the term *plurality coordination* (supportive social contexts coordinating plural logics) as a mechanism for individuals to organize conflicting medical logics and utilize them for their benefit (2017, 4).

Shim's concept of plurality coordination could add to an effective framework that addresses the tension between traditional health and biomedical practitioners and to develop a strategy for an alliance between the two medicines in the South African public health system.

CONCLUSION

Addressing the misalignment between different paradigms and practices of South African health care provision and the beliefs and desires of PWH utilizing this health care will take substantial global health and country-level political will and commitment, as well as a more thorough, critical, and self-reflective examination of the current practice of global public health. Achieving synergy between TAM and biomedicine will also require agreement on power sharing by the biomedical system. Shifting toward a culturally relevant, people-centered health care service based on a collaborative model of alliance and plurality coordination could provide a viable path to address the biopolitics of HIV/AIDS and balance the power dynamics that have been detrimental to the ultimate goal of the main two actors of the South African plural health system, improving the health and well-being of their patients.[5]

NOTES

1. Reflexivity Statement: The content of this chapter is directly influenced by my personal and ethnographic experiences taking place in the country of South Africa starting in 2004. From 2009 until 2018 I spent one to two months per year in the South African Province of KwaZulu-Natal. These experiences were framed by a context of collaborative anthropological and biomedical research on biomedical HIV treatment and health care provision and their intersection with TAM practices in KwaZulu-Natal. My positionality in these experiences has been informed by very salient aspects of my identity such as gender (I identify as a cisgender, heterosexual woman), skin color and ethnicity (I am a light-skinned Latina from Colombia, South America); my academic background and professional context (anthropology, medical anthropology, and public health); and my socioeconomic, professional, institutional, and residential statuses (a middle-class academician who lives in the United States and has an a formal association with an institution of higher education from the United States). Currently, I make part of

a multinal-national (South Africa/United States/Europe) biomedical and public health research team conducting implementation science in South Africa.

2. Cosmology is used here in its anthropological meaning, as the various notions that different cultures have about the way the world works.

3. Virologic failure occurs when ART fails to suppress and sustain a person's viral load.

4. The isiZulu term Makhosi has two meanings: a greeting to a person and her/his ancestors or, as in the context of this quote, a title for someone that is a traditional healer or THP.

5. I would like to sincerely thank the many HIV patients and traditional and biomedical health practitioners that have participated in our research in South Africa throughout the past decade, as well as my colleagues, both in South Africa and the United States. I am very grateful for all that I have learned from everybody. I would like to especially thank the following friends and colleagues in South Africa: Dr. Henry Sunpath, Dr. Christina Edwin, Dr. Jaysingh Brijkumar, Dr. Yunus Moosa, Mr. Selvan Pillay, Dr. Sally John, Pastor Sifiso Shange, Dr. Eleanor Preston-Whyte, Dr. Jane Hampton, Dr. Helga Holst, Dr. Krista Dong, Mr. Jasper Hansen, Mrs. Deli Mthimkhulu, Mr. Sandile Hlongwane, Ms. Mary Dong, and the staff of iTEACH and the RFVF Project. Many thanks to Dr. Diana Jeang, Ms. Dina Pimenova, Dr. Kimbi Hagen, Ms. Pam Eidson, Ms. Hannah Appelbaum Belisle, Dr. Monique Hennink, and Dr. Vincent Marconi in the United States. Last but not least, I want to thank my family for all the support. Special thanks to my parents and my husband, Vince, and children, Daniel and Alessandra. I could not have done any of this work without your loving support.

REFERENCES

Abdool Karim, Quarraisha, and Salim S Abdool Karim. 2002. "The evolving HIV epidemic in South Africa." *International Journal of Epidemiology* 31(1), (February): 37–40. https://doi.org/10.1093/ije/31.1.37.

Appelbaum Belisle, Hannah, Monique Hennink, Claudia E. Ordóñez, Sally John, Eunephacia Ngubane-Joye, Jane Hampton, Henry Sunpath, Eleanor Preston-Whyte, and Vincent C. Marconi. 2015. "Concurrent Use of Traditional Medicine and ART: Perspectives of Patients, Providers and Traditional Healers in Durban, South Africa." *Global Public Health*, 10(1), 71–87. https://doi.org/10.1080/17441692.2014.967709

Avert. 2020. "HIV Treatment Programmes Overview" Avert.org, Global Education and Information on HIV and AIDS. Updated 15 April 2020. https://www.avert.org/professionals/hiv-programming/treatment/overview.

Baker, Aryn. 2019. "What South Africa Can Teach Us as Worldwide Inequality Grows." *TIME*, May 2, 2019. https://time.com/longform/south-africa-unequal-country/.

Biehl, João, and Adriana Petryna, eds. 2013. *When People Come First: Critical Studies in Global Health*. Princeton: Princeton University Press.

Bordin, Edward S. 1979. "The generalizability of the psychoanalytic concept of the working alliance." *Psychotherapy: Theory, Research and Practice,* 16(3), 252–60. https://doi.org/10.1037/h0085885.

Cloete, Christie, Susan Regan, Janet Giddy, Tessa Govender, Alison Erlwanger, Melanie R. Gaynes, Kenneth A. Freedberg, Jeffrey N. Katz, Rochelle P. Walensky, Elena Losina, and Ingrid V. Bassett. 2014. "The Linkage Outcomes of a Large-Scale, Rapid Transfer of HIV-Infected Patients from Hospital-Based to Community-Based Clinics in South Africa." *Open Forum Infectious Diseases*, 1(2), (Summer 2014). https://doi.org/10.1093/ofid/ofu058.

Decoteau, Claire Laurier. 2013. *Ancestors and Antiretrovirals: The Biopolitics of HIV/AIDS in Post-Apartheid South Africa*. Chicago and London: University of Chicago Press.

Fassin, Didier, and Helen Schneider. 2003. "The Politics of AIDS in South Africa: Beyond the Controversies." *The BMJ*, 326(7387), 495–97. https://doi.org/10.1136/bmj.326.7387.495.

Flint, Karen. 2008. *Healing Traditions: African Medicine, Cultural Exchange, and Competition in South Africa, 1820–1948*. Athens: Ohio University Press.

Gona, Philimon N., Clara M. Gona, Suha Ballout, Sowmya R. Rao, Ruth Kimokoti, Chabila C. Mapoma, and Ali H. Mokdad. 2020. "Burden and changes in HIV/AIDS morbidity and mortality in Southern Africa Development Community Countries, 1990–2017." *BMC Public Health* 20(867) (2020). https://doi.org/10.1186/s12889-020-08988-9

Hammond-Tooke, William David. 1989. *Rituals and Medicines: Indigenous Healing in South Africa*. Johannesburg: Ad Donker.

Hansoti, Bhakti, George Mwinnyaa, Elizabeth Hahn, Aditi Rao, John Black, Victoria Chen, Kathryn Clark, William Clarke, Anna L. Eisenberg, Reinaldo Fernandez, Joshua Iruedo, Oliver Laeyendecker, Roshen Maharaj, Pamela Mda, Jernelle Miller, Nomzamo Mvandaba, Yandisa Nyanisa, Steven J. Reynolds, Andrew D. Redd, Sofia Ryan, David F. Stead, Lee A. Wallis, and Thomas C. Quinn. 2019. "Targeting the HIV Epidemic in South Africa: The Need for Testing and Linkage to Care in Emergency Departments." *EClinical Medicine*, 15, 14–22. https://doi.org/10.1016/j.eclinm.2019.08.007.

Hodes, Rebecca. 2018. "HIV/AIDS in South Africa." *Oxford Research Encyclopedia of African History*. https://doi.org/10.1093/acrefore/9780190277734.013.299.

Human Sciences Research Council (HSRC). 2018. "HIV Impact Assessment Summary, July 2018." *The Fifth South African National HIV Prevalence, Incidence, Behaviour and Communication Survey, 2017: HIV Impact Assessment Summary Report*. Cape Town: HSRC Press.

International Monetary Fund. 2020. "South Africa: 2019 Article IV Consultation-Press Release; and Staff Report; and Statement by the Executive Director for South Africa." *IMF Staff Country Reports*. International Monetary Fund, Country Report No. 20/33. January 30, 2020.

Katz, Ingrid T., Ingrid V. Bassett, and Alexi A. Wright. 2013. "PEPFAR in Transition—Implications for HIV Care in South Africa." *The New England Journal of Medicine*, 369(15), 1385–7. https://doi.org/10.1056/NEJMp1310982.

Kive, Paul. 2006. "Guidelines for Being Strong White Allies." Adapted from *Uprooting Racism: How White People Can Work for Social Justice*." www.paulkivel.com https://www.racialequitytools.org/resourcefiles/kivel3.pdf.

Krebs, Emanuel, Benjamin Enns, Linwei Wang, Xiao Zang, Dimitra Panagiotoglou, Carlos Del Rio, Julia Dombrowski, Daniel J. Feaster, Matthew Golden, Reuben Granich, Brandon Marshall, Shruti H. Mehta, Lisa Metsch, Bruce R. Schackman, Steffanie A. Strathdee, and Bohdan Nosyk. "Developing a Dynamic HIV Transmission Model for 6 U.S. Cities: An Evidence Synthesis." *PLoS One* 14(5), e0217559. https://doi.org/10.1371/journal.pone.0217559.

Mabaso, Musawenkosi, Lehlogonolo Makola, Inbarani Naidoo, Lungelo Lethukuthula Mlangeni, Sean Jooste, and Leickness Chisamu Simbayi. 2019. "HIV Prevalence in South Africa through Gender and Racial Lenses: Results from the 2012 Population-Based National Household Survey." *International Journal for Equity in Health*, 18(1), 167. https://doi.org/10.1186/s12939-019-1055-6.

Macciocchi, Stephen. "Doing Good: The Pitfalls of Beneficence." *Journal of Head Trauma Rehabilitation.* January/February, 24, 1 (2009), 72–4.

Malakoane, B., J. Christo Heunis, Perpetual Chikobvu, Nanteza Gladys Kigozi, and Willem H. Kruger. 2020 "Public Health System Challenges in the Free State, South Africa: A Situation Appraisal to Inform Health System Strengthening." *BMC Health Serv Res* 20, 58 (2020). https://doi.org/10.1186/s12913-019-4862-y

Malan, Mia, Dylan Bush, and Danny Booysen. 2019. "Growing up in the time of HIV: 'The babies we saved from HIV decades ago are now contracting the virus in their teens'" *Bhekisisa Centre for Health Journalism, South Africa.* Podcast, September 18. https://bhekisisa.org/multimedia/2019-09-18-podcast-growing-up-in-the-time-hiv-the-babies-we-saved-from-hiv-decades-ago-are-now-contracting-the-virus-in-their-teens/.

Mallett, Rich. 2014. "Where Do People Go When They're Sick? Traditional Healers Versus Modern Clinics in Sierra Leone." *Slate.* October 3. https://slate.com/technology/2014/10/sierra-leone-plural-health-care-system-why-people-go-to-traditional-healers-rather-than-modern-clinics-photos.html.

Maphumulo, Winnie T., and Busisiwe R. Bhengu. 2019. "Challenges of Quality Improvement in the Health care of South Africa Post-Apartheid: A Critical Review." *Curationis*, 42(1), e1–e9. https://doi.org/10.4102/curationis.v42i1.1901

Meyer-Rath, Gesine, Leigh F. Johnson, Yogan Pillay, Mark Blecher, Alana T. Brennan, Lawrence Long, Harry Moultrie, Ian Sanne, Matthew P. Fox, and Sydney Rosen. 2017. "Changing the South African National Antiretroviral Therapy Guidelines: The Role of Cost Modelling." *PLoS One*, 12(10), e0186557. https://doi.org/10.1371/journal.pone.0186557.

Mokgobi, Maboe G. 2013. "Towards Integration of Traditional Healing and Western Healing: Is This a Remote Possibility?" *African Journal for Physical Health Education, Recreation, and Dance* (Suppl 1), 47–57.

Moshabela, Mosa, Thembelihle Zuma, Joanna Orne-Gliemann, Collins Iwuji, Joseph Larmarange, and Nuala McGrath, and the ANRS 12249 TasP Study Group. 2016. "It Is Better to die": Experiences of Traditional Health Practitioners within the HIV Treatment as Prevention Trial Communities in Rural South Africa (ANRS 12249 TasP trial)." *AIDS Care*, 28 (Suppl 3), 24–32. https://doi.org/10.1080/09540121.2016.1181296.

Mothibe, Mmamosheledi E., and Mncengeli Sibanda. 2019. "African Traditional Medicine: South African Perspective." In *Traditional and Complementary Medicine*, Edited by Cengiz Mordeniz. DOI: 10.5772/intechopen.83790.

Ordóñez, Claudia E., and Vincent C. Marconi. 2012. "Understanding HIV Risk Behavior from a Sociocultural Perspective." *Journal of AIDS and Clinical Research*, 3(7), e108. https://doi.org/10.4172/2155-6113.1000e108.

Oseni, Zainab, and Geordan Shannon. 2020. "The Relationship between Indigenous and Allopathic Health Practitioners in Africa and Its Implications for Collaboration: A Qualitative Synthesis." *Global Health Action*, 13(1), 1838241. https://doi.org/10.1080/16549716.2020.1838241.

Peltzer, Karl. 2009. "Traditional Health Practitioners in South Africa." *The Lancet*. 374 September 19, 2009. doi:10.1016/S0140-6736(09)61261-7.

Pimenova, Dina. 2019. "The Viability of a Partnership between Traditional Health Practitioners and the South African Health care System: A Qualitative Systematic Review." Thesis Manuscript, Rollins School of Public Health, Emory University. Unpublished.

Sangaramoorthy, Thurka. 2018. "Chronicity, Crisis, and the 'End of AIDS'." *Global Public Health,* 13(8), 982–96. doi 10.1080/17441692.2018.1423701

Shim, Jae-Mahn. 2017. "The Coordination of Plural Logics of Action and Its Consequences: Evidence from Plural Medical Systems." *PLoS One*, 12(12), e0189841. https://doi.org/10.1371/journal.pone.0189841.

Statistics South Africa. 2012. "Census 2011: Census in Brief." Pretoria: Statistics South Africa. http://www.statssa.gov.za/census/census_2011/census_products/Census_2011_Census_in_brief.pdf.

South African Government. 2007. "Traditional Health Practitioners Act 22 of 2007." Republic of South Africa. https://www.gov.za/documents/traditional-health-practitioners-act.

South African Government. 2018. "Brand South Africa on HIV and World AIDS Day." Republic of South Africa. https://www.gov.za/speeches/brand-south-africa-calls-citizens-get-tested-hiv-and-know-their-status-world-aids-day-1-dec.

UNAIDS. 2007. "Traditional Healers Join the AIDS Response." UNAIDS. https://www.unaids.org/en/resources/presscentre/featurestories/2007/february/20070207traditionalhealersbp.

UNAIDS. 2020. "Country: South Africa." https://www.unaids.org/en/regionscountries/countries/southafrica.

Yamey, Gavin, Jesper Sundewall, Helen Saxenian, Robert Hecht, Keely Jordan, Marco Schäferhoff, Christina Schrade, Cécile Deleye, Milan Thomas, Nathan Blanchet, Lawrence Summers, and Dean Jamison. 2016. "Reorienting Health Aid to Meet Post-2015 Global Health Challenges: A Case Study of Sweden as a Donor." *Oxford Review of Economic Policy* 32(1), 122–46. https://doi.org/10.1093/oxrep/grv024.

Zuma, Thembelihle, Daniel Wight, Tamsen Rochat, and Mosa Moshabela. 2018. "Navigating Multiple Sources of Healing in the Context of HIV/AIDS and Wide Availability of Antiretroviral Treatment: A Qualitative Study of Community Participants' Perceptions and Experiences in Rural South Africa." *Frontiers in Public Health*, 6, 73. https://doi.org/10.3389/fpubh.2018.00073

Chapter 5

Who's Positive and Healthy Enough in West Africa for an Ebola Clinical Trial?

Oumy Thiongane and Janice Graham

The biocapital of drug and vaccine development, while fueling important innovations, can also stoke structural inequities in disease transmission, first providing resources but then taking them away when attention disappears (Graham 2001; Bibeau, Graham and Fleising 2006; Sunder Kaushik 2006).[1] Health system strengthening through resourcing public health, disease surveillance, detection and tracing in communities, and open science collaborations to develop vaccines and treatments gain the attention of governments during epidemics. International agreements are signed but then forgotten in a political turn until the next emergency (e.g., WHO International Health Regulations 2005/ 2019). Filovirus[2] laboratories, established after the discovery of Ebola virus disease (EVD) in Zaire in 1976, were abandoned by the next generation of scientists studying human immunodeficiency virus (HIV) (David, Nakouné and Giles-Vernick 2020), leaving Ebola researchers to scramble for another space for their research. Ebola, a disease that primarily kills Africans in small remote communities far away from the interest of world economies, sat in the shadow of the exceptional AIDS pandemic that started sweeping the world in 1983, killing millions. Within a week of the 2014 declaration of the Ebola Public Health Emergency of International Concern, however, billions of dollars of funds began rolling in to reactivate the development of Ebola vaccines. Had Ebola affected wealthy nations, there is little doubt that a vaccine would have been developed a decade sooner (Graham 2019), as multiple COVID-19 vaccines are under development currently. In the ebb and flow of global health drug development and financialization, funding for Ebola research faded with the explosion of HIV in the Global North and returned only when it became a global threat beyond Africa.

Adia Benton and colleagues' critical work on HIV exceptionalism, the biopolitics of positive health, and the neoliberal framing of quality of life of people living with HIV (Benton 2015; Benton, Sangaramoorthy and Kalofonos 2017) calls on researchers to consider the confluence of emerging diseases with the health technologies that cure, treat, or prevent them. Clinical trial research is central to that work. For anthropologists on the ground during the West African Ebola outbreak (2013–2016), it is difficult not to compare Ebola viral disease[3] with HIV in its earlier years. Sufferers of these infectious diseases have been heavily stigmatized, with temporal and spatial displacements that signal race (i.e., the portrayal of Ebola as an exceptional acute African disease; HIV as a now normalized chronic African disease). Their disease course and sufferers' experiences have been intimately affected by health care and technology innovations. While at the start of both the HIV and Ebola outbreaks, infection meant death, as research and response were mobilized, survival improved for those fortunate enough to be in the right place at the right time. Any treatment and care beyond none at all can be deemed exceptional. Those surviving Ebola or living with HIV continue to undergo scrutiny of the biomarkers and parameters of their healthiness.

The social, political, economic, geographical, and biological spaces of PLHIV are rarely considered by the clinical trial researchers who recruit them as study subjects. Variability in time and place across research sites that span countries and continents is largely taken for granted. And yet the people recruited for international, multisited clinical trials from distant countries are as diverse as the places in which they live and labor. To counter, instead of acknowledging difference, clinical research requires that study protocols, methods, and measurements meet standard operating procedures, regardless of their local appropriateness. Focusing primarily on one West African clinical trial site, WASite1,[4] this chapter explores what it meant to *be HIV+ and healthy enough* in West Africa in order to participate in a vaccine clinical trial for Ebola. What relevance does an experimental Ebola vaccine have for the everyday lives of HIV+ West Africans volunteering to participate in an Ebola trial?

THE CANADIAN AFRICAN TRIAL FOR AN EBOLA VACCINE (CATEBOLA)

Our ethnographic research team followed the standardizing process of an international Phase 2 Ebola vaccine clinical trial taking place in sub-Saharan Africa and Canada between 2017 and 2019. The Canadian African Trial for an Ebola vaccine (CATEbola) was a multisited double-blind, randomized controlled trial (RCT) involving five cohorts of PLHIV, 50 people in each cohort, whose inclusion was determined by their CD4 count.[5] The CATEbola study aimed to determine the safety and immunogenicity[6] of an experimental Ebola vaccine in HIV+ immunocompromised individuals. Initially, recruitment to Cohort 1 was to begin in Canada for healthy adults with HIV and a CD4 count of 500 or higher. The trial was then to travel to the African sites, where the trial investigators reasoned that more subjects with lower CD4 counts would be available.[7] A centralized computer-generated random allocation across all study sites, proportioned 4:1, determined whether a study participant was assigned the experimental vaccine or placebo.

First registered on clinicaltrials.com in December 2016, the CATEbola study was delayed by 18 months due in part to difficulties recruiting the Canadian cohort (David, Mathiot, Thiongane and Graham 2021). Beginning with "healthy" participants with an undetectable viral load (Cohort 1), the study aimed to finish with participants with a CD4 count greater than or equal to 200 (Cohort 4 [adolescents] and Cohort 5 [two-dose regimen of adolescents and adults]).[8] With the healthy participants in Canada only trickling in slowly, the trial team opened Cohort 1 to "healthy" HIV+ individuals at the African sites in mid-2018.

AN ETHNOGRAPHIC STUDY OF A CLINICAL TRIAL

Our ethnographic engagement with CATEbola at WASite1 took place over 14 months.[9] The numerous protocol, administrative, and financial amendments that had delayed the start of the clinical study also affected our ethnographic project, an independent study with its own funding, accountability, responsibilities, and scheduling that resulted in our having to leave the field at completion of Cohort 3. Still, we were able to observe the training sessions of trial staff, informed consent process, attend screening and vaccination sessions, medical consultations, home visits, team meetings and selected meetings of clinicians, and conduct interviews with clinical trial staff and study participants.

After the initial recruitment delays in Canada, the sites were permitted to recruit until each cohort quota of 50 participants was attained.[10] Any site's faster recruitment of a cohort necessarily resulted in fewer participants for that cohort needed from the other sites. This change in protocol sparked an unofficial competition between the two African sites who were motivated by a payment scheme that remunerated per participant; the more people recruited, the more resources could be requested from the study headquarters in Canada and allocated to that site.

Our ethnographic team conducted extensive observations at different locations, including the research center, local hospital, and in the community, completing 27 semistructured interviews with trial staff and participants.[11] Simultaneous notes were taken, as well as the sociodemographic data of the participants, some of whom became familiar to us through home visits or meetings in other locations. Contextually richer ethnographic opportunities emerged during these informal conversations.

DOUBLE STIGMAS: WHY WOULD SOMEONE WITH HIV WANT TO PARTICIPATE IN AN EBOLA TRIAL?

Our research explored why people with HIV would want to participate in an Ebola clinical trial. We wondered how the temporalities and localities of PLHIV shape a research study, and how the temporalities and localities of an international standardized trial shape study participants with HIV. The West African Ebola outbreak had created a unique opportunity to clinically trial candidate Ebola vaccines. The successful Guinea WHO "Ebola ça suffit" ring study, for example, was designed as an open-label cluster trial to vaccinate the ring of contacts around Ebola-infected people (Ebola ça suffit ring vaccination trial Consortium 2015; Henao-Restrepo 2017). That research design adapted the typical gold standard for a RCT that would have required blinding and a placebo control cohort, in order to meet the emergency needs of the epidemic. After the Guinea trial though, evidence from gold standard RCTs was required to license the vaccine, including further study of potentially vulnerable groups (e.g., children, pregnant, immunocompromised). CATEbola was one such clinical trial that would contribute to the data needed to license the Ebola vaccine. Unlike Guinea, which suffered considerable mortality during the outbreak, none of the three countries where the CATEbola trial was conducted were directly affected by the 2013–2016 West African or 2018–2020 Democratic Republic of Congo Ebola outbreaks.

Very few clinical studies describe the interaction between HIV and Ebola in patients (Purpura et al. 2017). Our ethnographic study of the CATEbola was intended to fill that gap. The participation of PLHIV in clinical research in West African settings is a missing piece in the history of antiretroviral therapies (ART) that centers on treatment, access, and equity. The World Bank, European Commission, United Nations Program on HIV/AIDS (UNAIDS), and pharmaceutical companies were at first reluctant to release expensive HIV drugs to low-income African countries. Reasons such as the procurement infrastructure and the incapacity of weak health systems to cope with drug resistance or potential adverse effects were cited, while Abstinence, Be Faithful, and use Condoms preventions were proposed. AIDS associations, activists, and citizen mobilization fought for greater access to drugs, price reductions, and the inclusion of patients in drug testing, including vulnerable populations whose disease burden and biological outcomes were affected by, for example, inequalities, racialization, and gender; eventually, people with HIV/AIDS became participants in clinical trials (Dalgalarrondo 2004). The West African initiative to access ART began in the early 2000s (Desclaux, Lanièce, and Taverne 2002; Hardon 2005). Multiple modes of access were debated, including user fees and technologies of confession that organized triage around those who could access and those who were left at the margins (Desclaux 2004, Nguyen 2010). As funding came to an end for these projects, however, PLHIV could no longer access resources from HIV programs, as they had dried up. Life became even more difficult for those without the power to sustain themselves. One CATEbola participant recounted:

> Before [referring to an association for PLHIV)] it was good . . . socially, having community meals, eating together. Outside, you feel stigmatized. In the association, you feel fulfilled because you are with your equals. Outside you don't have the right to drink from the same cup as others if you're infected. But once in the association, everything is allowed. Community meals help a lot of people, the orphaned children, their grandparents. We know that with the infection, we must eat well. Especially children. There were home visits . . . kits for home visits. Leading an activity, you do not feel embarrassed because you add a plus. But after, all these funds are blocked.

At WASite1, most trial participants were middle-aged women with dependent children and few resources. More than half were single or widowed; most of the married women said they were neglected by their husbands, some of whom had taken new wives. HIV/AIDS in this country is perceived to be more common in women, with men often denying their HIV+ status and refusing to support their infected wives. Women are left to continue without their husband's support. Participation in the Ebola clinical trial provided an avenue for some independence and employment, however minimal. Trial participation empowered these neglected women with HIV, and it gave them the opportunity to contribute to their children's lives and school fees after their husbands had died or taken new wives. For these women, hope was in their children and being able to look after them.

For CATEbola study participants at WASite1, Benton's concept of "living positively" was not evident. Immediate concerns centered around finding work and enough food to feed their children; being HIV+ was associated with having the biomedical markers of CD4, creatinine, and so on, for healthy clinical trial work; CD4 mapped to CD$. Tensions concerning the category of "healthy" in the trial study began early. Although the clinical trial promoted the health markers and rhetoric of what positive living is or should be, our fieldwork discovered considerable unrest with them. Positive living did not map to the adoption of the kinds of globalized moral, social, and physical practices for healthier living that Benton (2017) described. Instead, in the CATEbola study, positive living circulated around how the study staff adjusted research participants' bodies through nutritional counseling, performed several biomedical screenings until the acceptable metric appeared, and imagined how PLHIV needed to live in order to satisfy the study inclusion criteria. The role of standardized biological markers for participant eligibility, and their construction and translation throughout the study, triggered considerable concern and critique from clinicians and staff. The markers of being HIV+ and healthy, featured in the study inclusion criteria (e.g., free of clinically significant health problems; effective contraception; avoiding shared needles, razors, toothbrushes, kissing; presence of febrile illness; and a host of baseline lab tests for alanine aminotransferase (ALT), aspartate aminotransferase (AST),[12] creatinine, hemoglobin, platelet count, urine protein, occult blood, glucose, etc.), brought attention to the social and biological vulnerabilities in the participants' lives.

HIV/AIDS IN CONTEXT

The West African country where WASite1 was located has a population nearing 20 million and an HIV prevalence estimated at 0.7% in adults aged 15–49 years. In 2019, 100,000 (1.9%) were living with HIV, including 9,800 children under the age of 15. Women had 1.5 times the prevalence of men, though the hesitancy of men to get tested affects confidence in these estimates. Approximately 2,700 people were newly infected in 2019, with a wide margin of error (1,800–4,200), and 3,100 deaths were recorded, including approximately 700 children (UNAIDS 2019).

The country is far from attaining the UNAIDS goal set for 2020 where 90% of infected people know their status, 90% are on antiretroviral therapy, and 90% have an undetectable viral load (UNAIDS, 2014). In 2019, 73% of PLHIV knew their status, with 67% of those were receiving ART. With an unknown number of people with suppressed viral loads on treatment, and only 18% on ART having an undetectable viral load, the country is far from achieving even moderate viral load detection (UNAIDS 2019). Nevertheless, considerable efforts in the fight against AIDS have been made since first reported in the country in 1986. At the end of the 1990s, it was the second most affected country in West Africa, with more than 50% of hospital admissions due to HIV overwhelming the health system. The government's implementation of HIV planning between 1996 and 2000, following their late recognition of AIDS as a social disease in 1995 (i.e., their recognition that the disease shaped social ties, ethical and political issues beyond biomedical dimensions), paved the way for institutional responses, of which the 2002 initiative for access to ART is the most important (Ouattara 2003; Sanou et al. 2008). With prevention of mother-to-child transmission since 2002 and ART made free by decree in 2010, the AIDS prevention strategy reversed the epidemic curve, averting an estimated 1,000 new cases a year, reducing the rate of infection, and routinizing AIDS response. But while such programs gained steps toward ending HIV/AIDS (UNAIDS 2019), their decline added new liabilities.

THE GIFT OF A CLINICAL TRIAL

Numerous anthropological studies have shown that hope for better care is the primary motivation for HIV patients to participate in research (Brives 2013; Le Marcis and Rouamba 2012; Nguyen 2010). Institutional structures put in place at research sites make it relatively straightforward for a clinical study team to recruit from an active registry of patients in the regional hospital for PLHIV where ART is dispensed and biomedical follow-up provided.

The initial briefing for potential recruits about the CATEbola study took place at the regional HIV hospital on a Monday morning. Thiongane's field-notes described the event:

> A young physician in a white gown walks back and forth between the room and the hospital wards, assisted by two female HIV peer counselors. It's 8:20 when the hospital staff decide to start the information about the clinical trial although some people have been waiting since before 7 am. There are 18 people in the room, which will grow to 24 by the time the meeting ends.
>
> The physician does not speak the local language of the region, he belongs to another ethnic group from the centre of the country. He explains the study in French, he says that it is good news that brings us together, it is not about any therapeutic failure in their health but about a study that looks at healthy people like them. He reassures the people that their medical history is fine, that the "news is good," they are in good health, which is the reason they were chosen and eligible for a study on a vaccine against Ebola. Before this announcement, the people in the room had received no explanation for being summoned, so suspense in the room is total. The doctor quickly gets to the heart of the matter, explaining the organization of the experimental clinical trial.
>
> The division of participants into study cohorts according to CD4 counts, from high to low, is explained at length. One of the HIV peer counselors, we name her

> Ingrid, takes over by translating the clinician's words from French to the main local language. She chews a kola nut imperturbably while leaning against the wall. Behind her, another HIV peer counselor measures the silence by nodding in agreement. Ingrid congratulates the participants for having been invited to this first meeting. The clinical trial's interest in them is testimony of their ART compliance.

The study is presented by the clinical research team as a "gift." Participant 14 recaps what she has heard, "It was this information that says that this is a study, that there is a vaccine that they are going to do, that those who are going to be retained, it will be good for them. That's what they made us understand." For some participants, getting the vaccine is "luck" independent of compensation of CAD $25 for each visit.[13] One participant explained:

> My hope, that the vaccine they said was against Ebola, if it turned out to be the right one I received, I thank the good Lord. Because they made me understand that you can have the vaccine but it may not be for Ebola. You can get the Ebola vaccine too. Anyway, it's a matter of luck if I can tell. You can say that the vaccine you got is for Ebola, but it can be the other way around.

An HIV peer counselor presented the CD4 as "soldiers" that help to defend the immune system. While waiting for the experimental vaccine in an observation room, one trial participant recounted the discovery of his HIV and viewed the improvement in his CD4 count as both biological and social capital, positively relational to his physician:

> All this is a long story, I found out my serology in 2010. I have healthy children, it was my first wife who infected me, she died. . . . I arrived at the hospital for the first time with a CD4 count of 10 and today I have a CD4 count of 350 (he tells me this with a proud and satisfied look on his face). . . . Now, my physician is like a member of my family. (Thiongane Fieldnotes Journal, March 2019)

RESHAPING CELLULAR LIFE: STANDARD AND ADJUSTABLE CD4 COUNTS

Biologically monitored throughout, the selection of participants based on their CD4 count took on different meanings and values at each stage of the study. Therapeutic citizenship, conferred by those with the authority to determine PLHIV eligibility, legitimized certain choices (Nguyen 2010). One study clinician suggested that a CD4 count above 500 served as both evaluative measure and safety catch, offering some form of guarantee for the researcher of the participant's safety due to their "ability to tolerate the vaccine." "Please don't worry, your participation should not expose you to any damage or compromise your health. Next week's screening will help to determine your CD4 level. This check is out of concern for the safety of the participants. The CD4 count >500 is an indicator of your body's ability to tolerate the vaccine" (Consent Record Observation Notes, September 2018). This curious explanation, while far from the rationale and real purpose of CD4 criteria (to determine how the vaccine performed when confronting different CD4 levels), gave CD4 different social meanings.

The term "safety," in the manner articulated by the clinician, represented an authoritative claim that patient safety is a priority. However, the clinician continued, "It doesn't really mean safety. It's really about making sure that participating, being vaccinated, won't be seen as harmful, and we have to make sure that everything is okay even after the participant has withdrawn. It's a moral commitment to [the patient]" (Consent Record Observation Notes, September 28, 2018).

CD4 counts operate as a central biological marker for the study clinicians, who claim that it indicates the healthy nature of the positive participant's life from the start and while they progress through the vaccine trial. The trial rhetoric that rewards exemplary biological lives based on a healthy CD4 count and viral load[14] is still hypothetical during this first meeting, as we will see.

Observations and interviews conducted with health care staff and patients who lived in the neighborhood but were not part of the clinical study suggest three major obstacles to detecting viral load in the health care centers. The first is the shortage of active agents to perform the biological analyses; the second is the lack of available human resources, stuck in interminable labor strikes; and the third, perhaps of greatest concern, is the lack of information about viral load that may have consequence for safe sexuality and reproduction. The first two obstacles come from structural constraints in resource-limited settings where insufficient health care funding affects human resources, infrastructure, supply chain, test costs, and other complexities (Usdin, Guillerm and Calmy 2010). The third obstacle pivots on power and appropriate communication of knowledge when undetectable viral load information is not conveyed by a physician to the PLHIV.

This lack of disclosure of viral load by health care workers to PLHIV, the keeping of this information as a secret, is commonplace. Gaining knowledge of one's viral load is dependent on a number of factors, including the PLHIV's level of education, the awareness of the role of ART in viral suppression, and the physician's beliefs and motivation. Some people know their viral load but may not be aware of what it means for their everyday life; many are not told and do not know. Among many health care providers, the sexuality of PLHIV is perceived as risky or even licentious, and no matter the viral load, PLHIV are seen as potential virological bombshells for the HIV-population. Doctors fear that PLHIV will not comply with their treatment in the face of an undetectable viral load, undermining the efforts of ART and increasing the risk of drug resistance. The widely held belief that African PLHIV lack responsibility for compliance (Benton, Sangaramoorthy, and Kalofonos 2017) is a reverse stigma that has circulated since the 1990s by pharmaceutical companies and international public health leaders, persisting among some health care workers (Fainzang 2014).

For the above three reasons, not only do viral load results typically remain "secret" but patient consultations, testing, and follow-up are becoming further spaced apart. External to the study, the diagnosis, care, and follow-up of PLHIV had been significantly disrupted between 2016 and 2018 due to political unrest, street protests, and labor and funding cuts that led to a hospital crisis in the country (Bonnecase 2019). At the present time (2021), medical consultation has largely been reduced to collecting one's ART and quickly leaving the clinic. PLHIV are not informed of their CD4 count or viral load, if these are even measured. While taking ART, ordinary PLHIV are largely unaware of any changes to their viral load or whether the drugs are effective, an exceptional detail of significant importance in the CATEbola study by contrast.

The two primary criteria for inclusion in the trial are biological (e.g., CD4 count) and clinical (physician) assessment. We observed, however, a tension between clinicians' objectivity and partiality, where clinical criteria can be ambiguously interpreted, especially dealing with comorbidities that are not considered detrimental to participation. Several such conditions were not listed in the study protocol but left to the discretion of the clinicians; most clinicians interviewed indicated they were uncertain what to do with hepatitis, dermatitis, eye problems, and other conditions that could mask potential adverse events following immunization with the experimental vaccine that had to be carefully monitored for the study. The study inclusion criteria are a case in point: "Absence of *clinically significant health problems that could affect patient safety, according to the investigator* after reviewing the relevant medical history and performing a clinical examination prior to entry into the study" (emphasis added). We discovered many different interpretations of "significant health problems" by the study site staff. For example, hepatitis B and C were not clinically significant for physicians at WASite1 but were for the Canadian site. Definitions of healthy clearly differed.

Participants were recruited from a hospital list, with patient profiles sent to the study site based on data from a hospital software program that proved to be outdated. In fact, during the first biomarker screening to verify inclusion criteria, clinicians realized that not only did some patients no longer have an undetectable viral load as claimed by the hospital triage and their records but some were in therapeutic failure. The vaccine trial therefore helped signal to the hospital the urgency of managing patients who were not exemplary "healthy" subjects as had been suggested in the information meeting for the vaccine trial.

Over time, as the trial began recruiting cohorts with higher viral loads, new challenges arose in participants meeting all the global biological criteria, such as for hemoglobin, platelet count, and total red blood cell count, as well as creatinine, protein, and glucose standards from urinary tests. Recruitment for Cohort 2 took significantly more time than expected and created further controversies at the clinicians' weekly meetings, where debates entailed over hematological values that defined the number of red blood cells required for patient inclusion (4,000) and the cellular values concerning the CD4 level (>350 and <500). In the absence of participants meeting these criteria, the option of repetitive screening (i.e., testing the same participant two or even three times) was applied, even though it was an expensive procedure.[15]

Tests were repeated to game normal fluctuations in individual biological values that were near the cutoff point due to a variety of known and unknown circumstances. A participant falling outside the recruitment range one day might meet eligibility criteria in another. Knowledge of what was needed to meet the retest requirements was applied; for example, since creatinine levels are affected by hydration, the hospital doctor, familiar with the profile of his patients, recommended that the potential participant's physician instruct them to drink more. In this way, an actual material measurable positive life reconditioning exercise took place during clinical meetings. The clinical study served to rearrange and adjust the required eligibility criteria of sick bodies. The staff description of this adjustment enterprise oscillated between concern and humor; the local goal was to go fast and recruit as many patients as possible who met the criteria established by the Canadian investigators, or another study site would get the payment for recruitment. The clinical trial was well situated in the Ebola economic landscape to biocapitalize weak bodies (Shepler 2017).

Jokes acknowledged that this biological fiddling was common at clinical study meetings, including comments about buying meat for those with low blood iron or providing targeted injections for those whose values needed boasting. At one such meeting, a doctor humorously suggested removing ART from a particular participant to lower CD4 counts and meet the cell values required for Cohort 2 enrollment. Thus, a double ambiguity was revealed—on the one hand, there were patients in poor condition whose biomarkers were below the norms or for whom new pathologies were discovered, and, on the other hand, the trial managers/staff never forgot their goal and therefore adjusted positive bodies to make them fit the experimental rationale (Brives 2015).

"THEY ARE SAYING THAT HIV IS JUST LIKE ANY OTHER DISEASE"

The normalization and routinization of HIV by study personnel, illustrated in the excerpts above, emanating from free access to ART since 2010, does not mean that HIV exceptionality has resolved issues of inconsistent health care for PLHIV and the fear and stigma that it still generates in this West African country. Being HIV+ is not accepted as normal in everyday life in the town where WASite1 is located. Clinicians do not disclose viral loads to their patients; HIV exceptionality is readily apparent and hardly positive (David 2019) except in its biometrics. During our exchanges with health care providers, they underlined that the decline in programs providing care to PLHIV and the lack of political will and stability have generated a complex array of situations: staff shortages, demotivation of health care personnel, rationalization of biological assessments, weak monitoring of the side effects of ART, a paucity of nonpharmacological interventions as well as options regarding pharmaceutical therapeutic replacements, therapeutic failure, lack of investigation of those lost to follow-up, and so on, were observed throughout our research. Most health providers in the public sector (general practitioners, lab biologists, radiologists, and dentists) gain their highest remuneration consulting in private clinics that provide quality service in much less overwhelming conditions than hospitals afforded. Private consultations provide significant additional financial resources for doctors, with public health sector salaries considered to be the lowest of the ECOWAS (Economic Community of West African States) countries after Togo. Demands from the heavily underfunded public health care sector, including the need to increase civil service salaries and upgrade career advancement, have sparked continuous health care labor strike actions throughout the country (Bonnecase 2019). As usual, wrestling between the medical sector and state has been felt most by those dependent on public health care.

In interviews, hospital staff and health care workers repeated that they were overworked; civil unrest associated with deteriorating work conditions have only hardened negotiations with the state. Continuous strikes become longer and longer, sick patients are refused care, evacuated from hospitals, and were observed participating in hospital sit-ins outside, without anywhere else to go. The hospital director acknowledged that this situation has led to an increase in inadequate follow-up of PLHIV. In this context, PLHIV are given the potential hope of benefiting from some improvement in their bodily health when they join an experimental community, such as CATEbola. Study tests might identify unknown conditions, treatments might be provided that are otherwise not, and an experimental vaccine may protect against a disease in an unknown future. For most, living with HIV is exceptional but hardly positive, stigmatization thrives, and not everyone can equally access treatment for the disease that most affects them.

CONCLUSION

HIV and EVD discourses dueled over protocol standards, normality, location, treatment, cure, prevention, and power. HIV exceptionalism, though hardly framed in neoliberal terms of positive health behaviors and not a part of everyday conversation, was written in the bodies with a common vernacular. If HIV is seen as becoming normal in global health discourses, it was clear from our fieldwork that caution should be lent to another, largely incomplete project in the Global South. Many PLHIV continue to experience deplorable stigmatization that prevents mostly the poorest from being tested, from knowing their status, or accessing the dwindling services of countries undergoing social turmoil, where political conflicts and displacement affect primarily women and children.

Silence, racism, and stigmatization are a harbinger in every plague and epidemic (Wright 2020). The tangible aspects of "positive living" noted by Benton and colleagues (2017) that involve disclosure of status to sexual partners, family, and friends; practicing safer sex; eating well; and access and compliance with medication assume secure conditions of well-being. The reassurances of this type of safety net are not evident in the lives of the CATEbola participants. HIV-AIDS stigmatization discourages such solace, and the lack of disclosure to many of their viral count challenges sexual relationships on multiple levels. Husbands deny their positive status; women join clinical trials secretly in defiance of their husbands to procure food, shelter, and security. At stake is how the political economy of the clinical trial compelled HIV bodies and behaviors to meet uniform eligibility criteria, procedures, and regimen—the standards of technoscience. Trial participants and their families' needs induced them to submit, commit, and present their bodies and blood to the vaccine trial. The small benefits of trial participation, such as the anticipation of medical care otherwise unobtainable in such a resource-strapped economy, were encouraging enough for participants to synchronize their bodies and behaviors to these criteria and to tolerate the regular extraction of their blood, despite the fact that it troubled them.

The Ebola vaccine trial researchers assumed, at the start, higher rates of HIV on the continent translated to its normality in Africa. They needed to find out if the vaccine would be safe and immunogenic for PLHIV there. But there is no taken for granted "normal" with HIV. Precarity, the need for remuneration and extra medical care, and doctor-patient relationships drove trial participation for those with cause to fear disclosure and despite double stigmatization in their society of Ebola and HIV. The Ebola vaccine was injected into the bodies of hundreds of thousands of Africans during the five years of international clinical trials and emergency use, leading up to its approval in late 2019. Of those who contributed a year of their lives to the CATEbola study, any positive benefits that came from participation, such as access to additional medical care, knowledge of therapeutic failure that would otherwise have gone undetected, and some additional economic resources, would hardly have been exceptional if the global promise of 90-90-90 treatment for all had been met.

NOTES

1. As anthropologists turned their ethnographic lenses to laboratories, technoscience and sociotechnical relations, the substantive inequalities promulgated by the instruments of capital markets and biopower, such as intellectual property, became evident. Studies of the sociotechnical relations circulating among discovery science and the laboratory, the pharmaceutical industry, venture capital, biocapital, regulatory cultures, and the like have become central to anthropological science and technology studies (Krautwurst 2021; Sunder Rashan 2012).

2. Filoviruses, such as Ebolavirus, Marburgvirus, and Cuevavirus, cause severe hemorrhagic fever in humans and nonhuman primates.

3. There have been 26 Ebola outbreaks in 10 African countries since it was first reported in 1976. The West African Ebola epidemic was the largest, infecting over 28,000 and killing nearly 12,000. Symptoms include fever, headache, nausea with vomiting, diarrhea, septic shock, hemorrhage, and multiorgan failure. It is highly infectious with an estimated 50% mortality rate.

4. The African countries remain anonymous to protect the confidentiality of study participants and clinical trial staff, and name of the clinical trial, the Canadian African Trial for Ebola Vaccine (CATEbola), is a pseudonym. The country where WaSite 1 is located was the second most affected in West Africa.

5. CD4 is an indicator of immune function in patients living with HIV. It is commonly taken in an initial assessment of in vivo antiretroviral drug activity and used as a surrogate marker for clinical outcome in antiretroviral therapeutic trials. Initially utilized in determining ART eligibility and time to initiate therapy, nowadays viral load (HIV RNA) and CD4 cell count are used in the monitoring of HIV/AIDS progression.

6. Immunogenicity is the ability of a vaccine to mount an immune response in the vaccinated individual, thereby protecting them from disease. It is central to the determination of a vaccine's effectiveness.

7. Cohorts 2 and 3 included adults with a CD4 > 350 and <500, and ≥ 200 and ≥ 350, respectively. Cohort 4 targeted adolescents with CD4 ≥ 200, while Cohort 5

(added later) included adolescents and adults with a CD4 >200 receiving two doses of the vaccine.

8. At the time of final submission of this chapter (April 2021), the clinical trial was on hold, not having completed Cohorts 4 and 5 due to COVID-19 pandemic measures to reduce all nonessential research activities and declining urgency for results after the vaccine was approved. Marketed as "Ervebo," the vaccine licensed by the US FDA on December 19, 2019, followed by the Democratic Republic of the Congo, Burundi, Ghana, and Zambia in February 2020.

9. Our ethnographic study was funded by the Canadian Institutes of Health Research (PJT-148908). Ethical approval was obtained from Dalhousie University and national and hospital ethics committees at the research sites in the three countries where the study took place.

10. Recruitment stopped when 75% of each cohort data was available, to allow the external Data Safety Monitoring Board to conduct safety monitoring analyses. When no adverse events were detected, recruitment could start on the next cohort.

11. Conducted in local languages and French, audio-recorded interviews were obtained after a deliberative informed consent process with participants; one audio was lost.

12. Blood tests for the enzymes ALT and AST are used to detect liver damage.

13. The study involved eight visits. Participants received reimbursement payments of $25 on days 3, 7, 14, 28, 42, and 365. They were compensated $4 for the visit involving signing the consent form. There was no compensation for screening visits despite the fact it might need to be repeated.

14. Viral load is another standard of care used to monitor treatment efficacy in the study. It is measured every six months when the biological reagent is available and staff are not on strike.

15. According to the study protocol, a participant could be retested twice.

REFERENCES

Benton, Adia. 2015. *HIV Exceptionalism: Development through Disease in Sierra Leone*. Minneapolis: University of Minnesota Press.

Benton, Adia, Thurka Sangaramoorthy, and Ipolitos Kalofonos. 2017. Temporality and positive living in the age of HIV/AIDS. *Current Anthropology* 58, 4: 454–76.

Bibeau, Gilles, Janice E. Graham, and Usher Fleising. 2006. Bioscience and biotechnology under ethnographic surveillance: Where do Canadian medical anthropologists stand? In *Medical Anthropology: Regional Perspectives and Shared Concerns,* edited by Francine Saillant and Serge Genest. London: Blackwell, pp. 3–22.

Brives, Charlotte. 2013. Identifying ontologies in a clinical trial. *Social Studies of Science,* special issue: A turn to ontology on STS? 43(3), pp. 397–416.

Brives, Charlotte. 2015 'Pour eux c'est seulement à propos de la mortalité', la production des données et ses conséquences dans le déroulement d'un essai Clinique. *Sciences Sociales & Santé,* 33(2), pp. 41–64.

Dalgalarrondo, Sébastien. 2004. *Sida : la course aux molécules*. Paris: Éditions de l'École des hautes études en sciences sociales.
David, Pierre-Marie, Benjamin Mathiot, Oumy Thiongane and Janice Graham (2021) Under consent: particpation of people with HIV in an ebola vaccine clinical trial in Canada. *BMC Medical Ethics* 22; 42: 1–8. https://bmcmedethics.biomedcentral.com/articles/10.1186/s12910-021-00606-6
David, Pierre-Marie, Emmanuel Nakouné, and Tamara Giles-Vernick. 2020. Hotspot or blind spot? Historical perspectives on surveillance and response to epidemics in the Central African Republic. *International Journal of Public Health* 65, 241–248.
Desclaux, Alice, Isabelle Lanièce, Ibra Ndoye & Bernard Taverne. 2002 L'Initiative sénégalaise d'accès aux médicaments antirétroviraux: Analyses économiques, sociales, comportementales et médicales. Agence nationale de recherches sur le sida (ANRS). https://www.anrs.fr/sites/default/files/2017-09/initiative_senegalaise_acces_arv_oct2002.pdf
Desclaux, Alice. 2003. Stigmatisation, discrimination: que peut-on attendre d'une approche culturelle? UNESCO. https://halshs.archives-ouvertes.fr/halshs-00079800/document.
FDA News Release. 2019. First FDA-approved vaccine for the prevention of Ebola virus disease, marking a critical milestone in public health preparedness and response. https://www.fda.gov/news-events/press-announcements/first-fda-approved-vaccine-prevention-ebola-virus-disease-marking-critical-milestone-public-health
Faizang, Sylvie. 2014. Les inégalités au sein du colloque singulier: l'accès à l'information. *Les Tribunes de la santé* 43(2) (15 juillet 2014), 47–52.
Graham, Janice E. 2001. Harbinger of hope or commodity fetishism: "re-cognizing" dementia in an age of therapeutic agents. *International Psychogeriatrics*, 13(2), 131–134.
Graham, Janice E. 2019. Ebola vaccine innovation: a case study of pseudoscapes in global health. *Critical Public Health* 29(4), 401–412. DOI:10.1080/09581596.2019.1597966
Hardon, Anita. 2005. La lutte contre l'épidémie de VIH/Sida en Afrique subsaharienne: les politiques à l'épreuve de la pratique. *Revue internationale des sciences sociales*, no. 4: 661–669.
Henao-Restrepo Ana Maria, Anton Camacho, Ira M. Longini, Conall H. Watson, John W. Edmunds, Mathias Egger, Miles W. Carroll, Nathalie E. Dean, Ibrahima Diatta, Moussa Doumbia, Bertrand Draguez, Sophie Duraffour, Godwin Enwere, Rebecca Grais, Stephen Gunther, Pierre-Stephane Gsell, Stéphane Hossmann, Sara Vikemoen Watle, Mandy Kader Kondé, Sakoba Kéïta, Souleymane Kone, Eewa Kuisma, Myron M. Levine, Sema Mandal, Thomas Mauget, Gunnstein Norheim, Ximena Riveros, Aboubacar Soumah, Sven Trelle, Andrea S. Vicari, John Arne Røttingen and Marie-Paule Kieny. 2017. Efficacy and effectiveness of an rVSV-vectored vaccine in preventing Ebola virus disease: final results from the Guinea ring vaccination, open-label, cluster-randomised trial (Ebola Ça Suffit!). *Lancet* 4, 389(10068): 505–518. doi: 10.1016/S0140-6736(16)32621-6. Epub 2016 Dec 23. Erratum in: Lancet. 2017 Feb 4;389(10068):504.
Krautwurst, Udo. 2021. "A Lab of One's Own": Entangled Measures and the Challenges of Redefining Standard-Lab Practice in Academic Context. In *The*

Social Life of Standards. Ethnographic Methods for Local Engagement, edited by Janice Graham, Christina Holmes, Fiona McDonald and Regna Darnell. Vancouver: UBC Press, pp. 46–62.

Le Marcis, Frédéric and George Rouamba. 2012. Trial and Routine: On the Problematic Relation between Routine Care and "Private Actors" within West-African Health Services (Burkina Faso). *Curare : Journal of Medical Anthropology* 36, no. 3: 211–226.

Nguyen, Vinh-Kim. 2010. *The Republic of Therapy: Triage and Sovereignty in West Africa's Time of AIDS*. Durham and London: Duke University Press.

Ouattara, Fatoumata. 2003. Les associations de personnes séropositives et la gestion du risque de stigmatisation à Bobo-Dioulasso (Burkina Faso). In *VIH/SIDA, stigmatisation et discrimination: une approche anthropologique*, 21–37. Paris: Unesco, 2003. http://www.documentation.ird.fr/hor/fdi:010070114.

Purpura, Lawrence J, Emerson Rogers, April Baller, Stephen White, Moses Soka, Mary J. Choi, Mahmoud Nuha et al. 2017. Ebola Virus RNA in Semen from an HIV-Positive Survivor of Ebola. *Emerging Infectious Diseases* 23(4), 714–715. https://doi.org/10.3201/eid2304.

Usdin, Martine, Martine Guillerm, and Alexandra Calmy. 2010. "Patient Needs and Point-of-Care Requirements for HIV Load Testing in Resource-Limited Settings." *The Journal of Infectious Diseases* 201, Supplement 1 (15 April 2010), S73–S77. https://doi.org/10.1086/650384.

Sanou, Marie Joseph, Barro Faustin, Cazal-Gamelsy, Robert, Geneviève Onadja, Ramdé Alphonse, Somda Antoine, and Nikiema Michel. 2008. Le programme national burkinabé d'accès aux ARV (2002–2008): bilan critique et perspectives. *Science et Technique. Revue Burkinabè de la recherche*, 2008, 51–63.

Shepler, Susan. 2017. "We know who is eating the Ebola money!": Corruption, the state, and the Ebola response. *Anthropological Quarterly* 90(2), 457–480.

Sunder Rajan, Kaushik. 2006. *Biocapital: The Construction of Postgenomic Life*. Durham and London: Duke University Press.

Sunder Rajan, Kaushik. 2012. *Lively Capital: Biotechnologies, Ethics and Governance in Global Markets*. Durham and London: Duke University Press.

UNAIDS. 2019. Country Specific Data, Burkina Faso https://www.unaids.org/en/regionscountries/countries/burkinafaso#:~:text=Burkina%20Faso%20%7C%20UNAIDS&text=There%20were%2094%20000%20%5B72,fall%20of%2046%25%20since%202010.

World Health Organization. 2005; 2019. Statement on the second meeting of the International Health Regulations (2005) Emergency Committee regarding the outbreak of novel coronavirus (2019-nCoV) https://www.who.int/news-room/detail/30-01-2020-statement-on-the-second-meeting-of-the-international-health-regulations-(2005)-emergency-committee-regarding-the-outbreak-of-novel-coronavirus-(2019-ncov)

Wright, Justin D. 2020. Hush-hush, a pale horse cometh: Mirabilis Manducat. Sapiens. https://www.sapiens.org/culture/hush-hush-a-pale-horse-cometh-mirabilis-manducat/?utm_source=SAPIENS.org+Subscribers&utm_campaign=98711be636-EMAIL_CAMPAIGN_2020_06_03&utm_medium=email&utm_term=0_18b7e41cd8-98711be636-182883737&ct=t()

Part II

ALWAYS NEVER NORMAL

POSITIVE LIVING IN "POST-CRISIS" TIMES

Chapter 6

"I can live a normal life"

Challenging Perceptions of HIV and (Re)productive Life in Japan

Pamela Runestad

> I was born with hemophilia, which can be a difficult illness to manage. When I received care for it in infancy, the blood products contained HIV and Hepatitis C so I was infected. . . . Health is about your body and mental health. Even if you have something, knowing you don't have to worry about being sick is part of health. I've been going to the hospital for treatment when I feel bad or am in pain for a long time. I think being able to live with your illness without worrying about being sick is part of health. To keep your health, eat well, sleep well, exercise . . . people with HIV need to manage their health carefully. They also need to make sure they don't have sexual intercourse without telling their partners about their status, get regular health checks, and take their medicine in addition to things like eating well, sleeping well, and exercising. . . . Laughing is also really important, and good for your immune system. In my own case, I was much happier after I got married and my immunity went up. Your mental health can really affect your physical health, so if you can laugh, be happy, it's important for your health. I think I'm healthy now. (Mr. Kawada, age 35, National Diet Member)

Mr. Kawada is one of the 30,000+ Japanese people living with HIV. Compared to countries where the new cases annually exceed Japan's cumulative caseload, and given his positive self-assessment, it may seem like Mr. Kawada is one of just a few and that Japan's HIV situation is relatively under control.[1] Combined with the fact that there is little attention to Japanese cases even within Japan, and that most Japanese efforts to curb HIV are focused overseas, it may not come as a surprise that the majority of Japanese people I interviewed in 2011 did not consider HIV/AIDS to be a domestic issue, and equated HIV with AIDS and death. This means that many Japanese picture non-Japanese people dying when they discuss HIV/AIDS. Furthermore, because Japan has a strong health care system, education system, and high rate of literacy, it would be easy to assume that the small number of Japanese people living with HIV are relatively well off. After all, Kawada himself says that he is "healthy now." Yet, Kawada's experience is one among many and not necessarily the norm (although men accounted for 95% of new cases in 2017, 75% of Japanese HIV+ men contracted it through sex with another man) (NIID 2017a,e,f).

In this chapter, I analyze the stories of five HIV+ Japanese men (*yōseisha*[2]) who contracted HIV in various ways. Their stories are demonstrative of the variations in infection routes and experiences related to these variations, challenging assumptions that Japan is homogenous, that HIV is not a domestic problem there, and that the socialized medical system could easily and equitably handle whatever cases might develop. These *yōseisha* narratives also illustrate how HIV experiences vary greatly due to when HIV was acquired: some became infected with HIV iatrogenically in the 1970s and 1980s when *yōseisha* were expected to die, while others were infected soon after the advent of antiretroviral therapy (ART), and one was diagnosed after the development of Highly Active Antiretroviral Therapy (HAART). All five cases, in different ways, demonstrate the ways in which the mainstream Japanese public has tried to frame HIV as foreign or a problem of "others" as a type of defense mechanism for the general public, and how *yōseisha* have grappled with the internalization of these ideas. But perhaps most importantly, these cases show how some *yōseisha* have strived to fit Japanese norms of everyday life despite assumptions in Japanese society that *yōseisha* could not fulfill familial or work obligations due to their HIV status or behaviors that led to their infection.

The interviews highlighted in this chapter were conducted as part of a larger project on HIV/AIDS in Japan from 2010 to 2011. The main objective of this project was to understand how people living in a privileged, resource-rich nation with a high rate of literacy and a socialized medical system experienced HIV. More generally, I was interested in how people living with chronic medical conditions, and a stigmatized condition in the case of HIV, described and aspired to health. In general, I found that Japanese people living with HIV struggled with some of the same basic issues about access and stigma found in differently privileged countries despite local assumptions that HIV was a foreign issue and not a domestic public health issue. In the course of my research, I attended a number of exhibitions related to HIV/AIDS, HIV/AIDS awareness events and parades, NGO volunteer trainings, and medical seminars. I also conducted interviews with *yōseisha*, medical professionals, infectious disease researchers, public health officials, and members of the general public. The research was multisited, and I worked in both rural and metropolitan areas across Japan.

HEALTH AND (RE)PRODUCTIVE LIFE IN JAPAN

Understanding the realities of *yōseisha* in Japanese society requires an understanding of how Japanese conceptualize health, and the importance of being a healthy person in Japanese society in terms of their ability to be a (re)productive person (a *shakaijin*). As I outline below, the general public imagines that being HIV+ makes a healthy life, and by extension life as a *shakaijin*, impossible—either because of the illness itself or because of the behaviors associated with infection.

Shakaijin—men and women—are valued for their productivity and reproductivity. Conservative Japanese politicians continue to espouse the belief that women raise future citizens as nurturers (and in some cases by working side or temporary jobs to supplement household incomes) while men contribute directly to the health of the nation through their workplace labor and the financial support it provides their families. Justification for adherence to these ideals is usually couched in terms of the plummeting birth rate and overall population decline in Japan, fears about the seemingly inevitable collapse of the Japanese pension system and other social supports, and in resistance to feminist assertions for the need for equal pay, daycare, and other forms of social support (Shigematsu 2015). Despite the difficulty of finding lifelong employment with a livable wage and benefits and the rising costs of raising children in Japan, young Japanese are still expected to pursue these ideals and are blamed for social problems when they do not (Coulmas 2008). In other words, productivity of men and reproductivity of women are considered to drive Japan's prosperity, according to aging (mostly male) politicians.

These core aspects of being a *shakaijin* are often linked to particular Japanese religious and philosophical influences. Although some scholars have drawn causative links between attributes of Japanese philosophical or religious practice and contemporary Japanese gender norms (see Hansen 2007 and Visscher 2006), few Japanese people identify as particularly religious or explain their behaviors in terms of these epistemologies. It is perhaps more accurate to say that the architects of modern Japanese society were influenced by Daoist, Confucianist, Buddhist, and Shinto ideologies, so they are "baked into" Japanese social institutions[3] (see, e.g., Sawada 2014) and have become part of what Stuart Hall calls primary culture.

It is equally important to consider that since World War II, both within and outside of Japan, the Japanese body politic is commonly presented as monolithic and undifferentiated, even though Japanese people are diverse according to region, age, socioeconomic status, education level, ethnicity, health status, gender, sexuality, and marital status, among other markers (Sugimoto 2003, Weiner 1997, Mackie and McLelland 2015, and Alexy and Cook 2018). The phrase "*ware ware nihonjin*" or "we Japanese" is often used to make generalized statements about what speakers imagine or wish to be true about the Japanese public (for a full discussion of Japanese exceptionalism, see Befu 2001), rather than reflecting an empirical reality. Living a "life according to the rules" (*kisoku tadashii seikatsu*)[4] or a "normal life" (*futsuu na seikatsu*) are variations on that theme in which the speaker conflates their own ideas and experiences of normalcy with their assumptions or beliefs about the behaviors and values of the rest of the population. Idealized gender norms (values and rules for being a man or woman) coalesce in the term *shakaijin*. The term literally translates as "person of society," but is understood to be a person who aims to contribute to society by becoming educated, getting a job, getting married, and having and supporting a family (Dasgupta 2006). In other words, being a *shakaijin* is part of being a good Japanese citizen and good health is linked to being able to take part in these rites of passage as a part of the "normal" life course.

The institution of marriage in Japan provides a useful example. In Japan, marriage is legally defined as being between a man and a woman, and many women are expected to leave their jobs either upon marriage or childbirth to manage the home and leave men with the job of wage earner (Borovoy 2005), meaning that "nontraditional" patterns of partnership and parenthood have little to no formalized social or financial support (Borovoy 2005, Alexy 2011). Women who engage in sexual behaviors outside the role of producing children within a marriage are considered "bad" women and threats to the body politic (Miller 2002; Miller and Bardsley 2005). Additionally, marriage partners may be chosen for pragmatic reasons rather than for attraction, making sex within marriage also pragmatic; thus, sexual intimacy may be conceptualized as something that happens outside of marriage. While Japanese people have been more likely to consider sex outside marriage as acceptable—even normal—it has been more socially acceptable for men than for women in the recent past (Allison 1994); more recent work has indicated that gendered expectations such as these may be shifting (Alexy and Cook 2018). Young Japanese—men and women alike—are also opting to get married later and have fewer children (ibid.).

Given these narrow parameters for defining what it means to be a "good" or "normal" Japanese person, sexual minorities are at risk of being stigmatized, particularly if they are open about their sexuality or decide not to marry or have children. From the standpoint of conservatives, such Japanese are not helping with the falling birth rate by marrying and having children. Although there is a long history of sexual diversity in Japan (Maree 2015, McLelland 2000 & 2005, Pflugfelder 1999, Leupp 1995), same-sex marriage is not legal, and nonheteronormative sex is marginalized and trivialized. For example, an interviewee in her 30s related the story of how she came out as lesbian to her mother in frustration because she had been pressuring her to get married: "My mother shouted back, 'being a lesbian has nothing to do with getting married!'" For her mother, marriage was about financial security and child-bearing regardless of sexual preferences, while the daughter sought emotional security from her partnership that is not grounded in dominant ideals about gender and sexuality. This young woman and her mother clearly viewed the relationships between marriage, gender, sex, and sexuality very differently, and demonstrate the ways that expectations about being a *shakaijin* are also heteronormative.

HIV+ or not, interviewees consistently discussed health in practical terms: being able to do "everyday things" like work, socialize, and move about the world unencumbered were valued, and being unable to do these things were points of anxiety. The idea of being a (re)productive member of modern Japanese society has been intertwined with assumptions about good health and fitness in order to successfully move through rites of passage such as employment, marriage, and childbirth under what conditions, making it ableist as well. During Japan's eugenics movement,[5] people with mental health conditions, leprosy, and other "undesirable" characteristics were forcibly sterilized (Robertson 2002; Fruhstuck 2003). More recently, Stevens (2007), Teruyama (2014), and Nakamura (2013) have described ongoing marginalization of differently abled individuals in Japan including people with physical differences, nonneurotypical individuals, and people with mental health conditions, noting that the embrace of idealized identities like being a *shakaijin*—which are tied to perceptions of health and "normal" bodies—is a barrier to diversity and inclusion efforts.[6] If a Japanese person has a chronic condition or is differently abled, they are rendered marginal to mainstream social norms and likely valued as a "less" vital member of society. Further, someone's health may suffer not because of their own situation, but because of other people's misperceptions of their health and abilities. In short, Japanese society is diverse in many ways, but the degrees to which that diversity is understood, catered to, and celebrated are limited.

Yōseisha must contend with wider social beliefs about their perceived inabilities linked to the assumption that having HIV is equated with AIDS and death, and therefore one cannot do the "everyday things" that make one a *shakaijin*. These assumptions include the belief that a *yōseisha* can longer work and will become increasingly disabled, making them an increasing burden on the medical system as they progress to AIDS. Another assumption is that *yōseisha* will not live long enough to care for their parents as they age, or perform rituals for their ancestors by managing the family altars or graves. A third assumption is that *yōseisha* have an infectious disease that has the potential to sicken and kill others, so if they marry and have children, they would spread the disease. Thus, according to these assumptions, *yōseisha* are not only incapable of providing the future generation of Japanese citizens, but they are a threat to the very existence of current and future generations due to the infectious disease they carry, and the supposedly "deviant" behavior that people assume caused them to be infected (such as sex work, drug use, or non-heterosexual sex).

These problematic assumptions make it difficult for *yōseisha* to meet *shakaijin* ideals. Nevertheless, many *yōseisha* still aspire to be *shakaijin* because the core values that are central to it—the importance of family, the relationship between individuals and society, and having a strong work ethic—are broadly shared values that are fundamental to being "a good Japanese person." Thus, despite assumptions to the contrary, many *yōseisha* view themselves as *shakaijin*. For example, all the *yōseisha* I met were employed. Some are married, have children, care for partners or aging parents, or take over the family business. All of the interviewees talked about the importance of staying healthy. They also talked about disclosure and safe sex, topics that never came up with my non-*yōseisha* interviewees even though they are critical to maintaining health and fertility. These *yōseisha* can and are engaging in these activities because that is what you do when you "live right"—HIV+ or not—as a *shakaijin*.

The first two cases I discuss below, when juxtaposed to those that follow, illustrate another set of important points: some *yōseisha* are viewed as blameless or innocent with regard to their route of infection because they were infected in utero or iatrogenically,[7] while others can be blamed for contracting HIV because of supposedly "deviant" sexual behaviors or drug use[8] that led to their infections. But even among so-called innocents, access to treatments and support networks is uneven, and this unevenness presents different challenges for those aspiring to be *shakaijin*.

IATROGENIC (*YAKUGAI*) INFECTION IN THE AGE OF EXPERIMENTAL TREATMENT: MR. KAWADA AND MR. TAMURA

In this section, I return to Mr. Kawada's opening vignette and contrast his experiences with Mr. Tamura's. Both of these men contracted HIV and hepatitis C as they received treatment for hemophilia. Iatrogenic infection, known as *yakugai eizu* in Japan, was the first "wave" of HIV/AIDS cases in Japan, and many died from AIDS complications before ART became available. Both men have been able to manage their three chronic illnesses due to medical advancements, but it is clear that knowing one has reliable access to cutting-edge technology *and* constant social support influences mental and physical health, making it more or less possible to fulfill one's aspirations of being a *shakaijin*.

Mr. Kawada is a politician in the National Diet of Japan.[9] He is a regular participant in public discussions of HIV. I met him at one of these events and later interviewed him at his office. Over fruit and tea, he related how he had contracted HIV and hepatitis C as an infant when he underwent treatment for hemophilia, and that his mother had told him about his HIV status at age 10. He lived part of his childhood and into his teenage years with this knowledge, and he learned about HIV through reading books and going to conferences with his mother-turned-activist from a relatively early age. Notably, he described himself as healthy and he told me that he has gone through many of the same rites of passage as his fellow Japanese constituents have: he went to university, got a job, and got married. His reliance on health maintenance—eating well, sleeping well, exercising, laughing—is very similar to what other Japanese have told me is essential to being healthy.

What is interesting about Mr. Kawada's account is his emphasis on not having to worry about getting sick. It is not just getting reliable treatment for all three conditions that help him maintain his health—it is knowing that it is there and not having to worry about having to seek it out. In almost the same way that automatic savings or retirement investments help build financial health, having a set team and regimen provides him peace of mind that if he does feel unwell, he has resources to use. In other words, worrying about his treatment is not a point of chronic stress. Although he may experience other forms of stress and/or chronic stress, not having to worry about this probably contributes in some measure to his mental health, which may then in turn contribute to his ability to foster relationships. Note the very different tone and experiences of Mr. Tamura:

> I have no memory of being told [about my condition] by the doctor. The thing I was most worried about at the time was what to do if my girlfriend had gotten it. When her result was negative, I was so relieved. For a while I thought I wouldn't live very long so I was consumed by desperation. On top of that, I was scared of what kind of discrimination and prejudice my family would face after I died. I decided I would go through life alone [not get married]. I lost my friends one after another. But after seeing (them die), this strong desire to live for them grew inside me.

> I was born in 1959. When I was a second year junior high school student [age 13, 1972] I went in for a hemophilia exam and had a blood transfusion. I lived a

normal life. When I was a first year university student [age 20, 1979], I started bleeding from my knees and had treatment [for hemophilia] for a year and a half. I was told I'd be in a wheelchair, and I left the university. I did rehabilitation until I could live as before, but in 1989, I started showing symptoms of AIDS. Miraculously, after three months of treatment, I could return to work. In 1995, I got interferon treatment for Hepatitis C. After one year, the virus disappeared but in 1996 I began showing symptoms of AIDS again and stopped working. In 1997 the AIDS Relief Center established the Habataki Project[10] and I have been a director since (14 years). I've known my HIV status for 25 years [since age 27, 1986]. Having HIV does not affect my ability to work and I've never had problems getting treatment. I've never been the victim of discrimination. The most distressing thing about having HIV is taking medications that cause strong side effects. The medicines we have now are a treatment, but you have to keep taking it. I would be extremely happy if we could develop medicine that you take for a set time that could completely heal you, and that you would never have to take it again. . . .

Being healthy means being able to use your five senses and go about everyday life. I've had this idea of health since 1972, when I was admitted to the hospital and I couldn't use my right hand for a half a year. Keeping healthy requires good communication with your doctors. I try to live a *kisoku tadashii seikatsu.*[11] I don't think I'm a particularly healthy person because there are a lot of difficulties in my daily life. (Mr. Tamura, age 52, Program Director)

Like Mr. Kawada, Mr. Tamura was infected with HIV and hepatitis C through blood transfusions for hemophilia in the 1970s. Unlike *yōseisha* who contracted HIV through sex or drug use, culpability for infection did not rest with Mr. Kawada or Mr. Tamura in the eyes of the public: blame was placed on practitioners and the Japanese government for failing to protect the blood supply even after it was known to be tainted (Seki et al. 2002). As *yakugai* cases, they have been able to avoid the judgment that other *yōseisha* who contracted HIV from sex face. Both men were treated with interferon and ARVs and have become accustomed to living with multiple incurable chronic conditions. Both had known their HIV statuses for 25 years at the time of the interviews, and both have worked to improve the lives of people living with HIV—Mr. Kawada through his work as a Diet member and Mr. Tamura through his work at Habataki. Furthermore, both men do share a status as "innocent" victims due to being infected through blood transfusions, and both aim to live a "*kisoku tadashii seikatsu*" by disclosing to sexual partners and taking responsibility for their health.

Despite these similarities, their definitions of health, assessments of personal health, and personal lives are very different. These differences are instructive because they show variation in *yōseisha* experience due to region, available resources, and time of diagnosis within the lifespan Mr. Kawada, who was diagnosed with HIV as a child, was able to gradually build his life with the knowledge that he was living with HIV, and went on to attend college, run for office, and get married. He has fulfilled many of the requirements to be a *shakaijin* in the eyes of the general public. On the other hand, Mr. Tamura learned about his status when he was 27 years old and had a girlfriend. Like many *yōseisha*, he thought he was going to die, and he described his fear and feelings of guilt that maybe his girlfriend had become infected, too. Even though she tested negative, they broke up and Mr. Tamura decided never to marry. Moreover, Mr. Kawada was raised by an activist mother who took him to meetings and conferences from the time he was a boy, while Mr. Tamura grew up in a rural area where he feared his family would suffer discrimination for his diagnosis. And although Mr. Tamura had been ill throughout his teens and 20s, he did not grow up with his HIV diagnosis the way that Mr. Kawada did. So although the two had known about their infections for about the same length of time, being diagnosed at different times in their lifespans and the particulars of their lives influenced the ways in which they experienced HIV. These particulars subsequently influenced the choices they made about family life and social engagement.

In contrast to the highly public venue where I first met Mr. Kawada (an HIV/AIDS forum in Yokohama) and where he asked his interview to take place (the government office where he worked), I met Mr. Tamura briefly at a café with some other acquaintances. He had come to a casual, nonresearch social gathering at the invitation of a mutual friend—one who knew Mr. Tamura's status and my research agenda. It was only after he left that I learned of his HIV status: he asked our friend to ask me if he could participate in my research by answering my interview questions on paper. I gave the blank forms to our friend, and the forms appeared in my mail slot, completed in Mr. Tamura's careful handwriting, about a week later. Our friend explained to me that he tired easily and thought writing was the best way to say what he wanted to say.

This difference in interaction is partially a function of personality, but it is also partially due to the very different settings and jobs these two men have. While Mr. Kawada lives in Tokyo, where there are a number of HIV specialists and organizations that cater to *yōseisha*, Mr. Tamura has lived in the same rural town all his life. There is one hospital where he can get care in the immediate area, and he works at the only office in town that caters specifically to *yōseisha*. While Mr. Kawada is a public figure with many connections to HIV/AIDS support groups, Mr. Tamura's circle of friends has shrunk: a number of his friends have died and, rather than seek a marriage partner, Mr. Tamura lives with a parent. In other words, Mr. Tamura has a more limited network of resources and social support in comparison to Mr. Kawada, and a more private life. Although he says he has not experienced discrimination as a *yōseisha*, I could not help but think that this may be because of the caution he exercises in social interactions, which helps protect him from exposure, stigma, and discrimination.

The two men talk about health differently, too. Mr. Kawada chose to discuss his happiness with me rather than past difficulties, but Mr. Tamura was blunt about the harsh realities of his life with HIV, including the fact that he has recovered from AIDS not once but twice. Additionally, Mr. Tamura had been confined to a wheelchair and had lost the use of his hand at different times. Based on what the two men shared with me, it seems that Mr. Tamura's physical health has been poorer than Mr. Kawada's. These differences may explain why Mr. Tamura described health as "being able to use your five senses and go about everyday life" while Mr. Kawada included "being able to laugh and be happy" as part of his definition of health, and why Mr. Kawada considers himself healthy while Mr. Tamura stated categorically that he is not. However, despite his feelings of ill health, Mr. Tamura noted that having HIV had not affected his ability to work. This may be aided by the fact that he worked for an organization that was created explicitly to support *yōseisha* (and people living with iatrogenic conditions in general).

Mr. Kawada's happiness and ability to feel free from worry with regard to his HIV status is the result of several factors that include his outgoing personality, education, profession, connectedness to his family and friends, and financial security. A portion of this happiness and apparent ability to be free from worry may be due to Mr. Kawada being fully open with his family, friends, and constituents about his HIV status. This level of openness about one's HIV status was absent in other *yōseisha* I interviewed. As someone who was infected through a medical treatment, Mr. Kawada is not blamed for his HIV status as are people who were infected through sexual contact or unsterile needles. That he was infected as an infant makes him a sort of "double-innocent." Not being judged about his status has made it possible for him to live as a public figure who happens to have HIV rather than live as a person defined by their HIV status. Rather than focusing on HIV status as a means to educate the public,[12] Mr. Kawada highlights his HIV status only when motivated or called on to do so, and feels that he is accepted by the public as someone with multiple roles and statuses.

Mr. Tamura's narrative demonstrates that, despite some similarities in transmission route, disease diagnoses, and illness trajectories, he does not feel the same openness as Mr. Kawada. Mr. Tamura was older and had a girlfriend when he found out that he was HIV+. He lives in a rural area with few HIV resources. He is, by his own account, shy and perhaps even more wary of people given his HIV status and his location. Many of his HIV+ friends have died from AIDS complications. He has struggled to regain and maintain his health, so his definition of health is shaped by extreme poor health experiences, such as the loss of the use of his legs. He also noted the ongoing reminder of ill health: daily doses of ART that he wished he did not have to take. Although he works hard and tries to be a dutiful son who takes care of his aging parent, he says there are many difficulties in his daily life. While he is able to access medical care, it is clear that he is not "free from worry" in the way that Mr. Kawada describes.

MSM INFECTION AND ART: HUNKY AND MR. SHIMATA

While Mr. Kawada and Mr. Tamura represent one risk group in the first wave of HIV patients in Japan, the vast majority of infections from the mid-1990s are a result of unprotected sex, and most recently between men who have sex with men (NIID 2017a). While iatrogenic infections from foreign blood products allowed the general public to consider HIV as foreign and Japanese hemophiliacs as victims, the increase of HIV in Japanese people through sexual transmission prompted the general public to focus on blame as a defense mechanism: if someone acquired HIV through sex, they had done something that was decidedly not "*kisoku tadashii*"—not according to the rules. For women, HIV was often couched in terms of sex with a foreigner or sex for goods or money (Miller 2002; Cullinane 2007; Runestad 2010). For men, it was couched in terms of sex with other men. Sex that resulted in disease and death and not healthy babies was perceived as threat to the body politic. While Mr. Kawada was a "double innocent" because of iatrogenic infection as an infant, *yōseisha* who contracted HIV from sex were doubly stigmatized—for their supposedly "dangerous" sex and for their HIV status. It was challenging for *yōseisha* who had internalized both the desire to be *shakaijin* and the discriminatory ideas about HIV and sexuality to navigate these aspects of their lives.

For all *yōseisha* I interviewed, ideas of personhood were strongly bound up with gendered, idealized expectations and obligations about family and work that are central to being a *shakaijin*. In the case of Hunky (a 60-year-old man diagnosed when he was 50), it was clear that it was coming out as gay and not as HIV+ that most complicated perceptions regarding whether or not they could fulfill familial expectations:

> What I was most distressed about when I found out my status was, "Why am I gay? Did I get HIV because I'm gay?" It took time to accept my own sexuality. And I'm married, right? I got married when I was 32. I was having sex with

women, too, at the time. Actually, I thought I was bisexual. But after I got married, I realized that I'm gay . . . accepting that took a long time. And telling my wife I was HIV+ took me a year and a half. That year and a half was necessary for me to accept that I was gay. So when I told my wife, I felt I had to tell her that I'm gay and HIV+ at the same time. When I told her, she said, "Well, we can keep on doing as we've been doing, right?" So—I'm married, but I'm gay. I'm positive, but my wife isn't. After I told her, I felt so much better. I'm not sure how she felt, but I was relieved.

It's harder to tell my parents that I'm gay than telling them I have HIV. . . . Sometimes people compare living with HIV in rural and urban areas, but I compare living with HIV in Tokyo and Osaka. In Tokyo, people come from everywhere, and you can be "free." But for me, my family all lives in Osaka and coming out for either thing is hard. Being gay is hard, harder than having HIV. When I was 18, it was like, where are the gay adults? There was no role model for us, for us as 30, 40-year old men with no families. I felt like I was going to die. Even the thought of making a baby was scary, because I was worried—what if my child is gay? I don't want them to have such a hard life. Now people are learning more about being gay, but still my brother and father think being gay is unimaginable.

I think to be healthy, you have to accept yourself. If you don't accept yourself, your body and mind can't be healthy. Before I got HIV, I didn't really think about it. Before, I thought if I didn't get sick I was healthy. But after I was infected with HIV, I had different experiences, and I realized that me just being alive was a great thing. I've known that I've had HIV since 2001. But if I were infected earlier, like five or six years earlier, maybe I wouldn't be here. Maybe I'd be dead. . . . When I first found out, there still wasn't a lot of information. I had to learn a lot about HIV and medicine, and at first I thought this is a terrible illness! And I was shocked. But now, I take medicine just twice a day and other than those times, I usually don't think much about HIV. It's just one part of me. (Hunky, 60, city employee)

Hunky is the "stage name" of a *yōseisha* who regularly speaks in public about HIV. He agreed to meet with me for an interview after one of these events. Despite his fears that his family will find out about his status or sexuality, he is a regular participant at public HIV/AIDS events and I heard him speak a number of times during my fieldwork (Runestad 2016). Hunky considered HIV a "terrible illness" when he was diagnosed. Prior to this, he had had a straightforward understanding of health as the absence of sickness. However, as Hunky learned more about life with HIV—that ARVs could help, for example—his ideas about health changed, too. More recently, being healthy has been predicated on accepting himself as gay and HIV+. Moreover, he says he has learned not to reduce his identity to his diagnosis or his sexuality. Neither of these facts has changed his marital status or his ability to work as a long-time employee at a city office near Osaka. What he has had to grapple with are the stigmas associated with being gay and HIV+ in Japan, stigmas that he had internalized at one point. In other words, what has been most challenging for Hunky hasn't been living with HIV, but rather society's misperceptions of nonbinary individuals and sexual minorities, which subsequently frame people's perceptions of HIV.

Hunky had learned of his HIV status 10 years prior to our conversation and has spent the past decade learning to live with HIV and accepting his sexuality. It may seem unusual that Hunky wanted to stay married to his wife once he realized he was gay and that the two opted to stay together once he disclosed to her, but these choices are largely protective for them and do not necessarily go against marriage ideals in Japan, especially for their generation. Although "love marriage" is fairly common among younger Japanese, it is not uncommon to consider marriage as pragmatic and to choose a stable partner who will be a good parent or provider instead of someone deemed attractive (Borovoy 2005). In other words, dependability may be a stronger factor than attraction in marriage, and sexless marriages (or ones that gradually become sexless) are not uncommon (Dales and Yamamoto 2018). Although Hunky and his wife do not have children, being married and employed make them "normal" in the eyes of the public and their families: they are upholding some (if not all) expectations of being *shakaijin*. If they had opted to divorce, they would likely face questions as to why, which would leave them with the choice to lie or to disclose Hunky's sexuality or HIV status or both. And even though his wife is not HIV+, this could make her vulnerable to discrimination. Moreover, Hunky was close to retirement age at the time of our conversation. Divorce and disclosure could also result in financial instability at the end of their prime working years.

Mr. Shimata is also a gay man in his 60s living with HIV. At the time of interview, he had been living with HIV for 25 years. He is unmarried and has some similar experiences to Hunky, but he tended to frame most of his experiences with HIV in terms of work. In our interviews (I met with him twice), Mr. Shimata did not mention self-blame for his diagnosis and did not seem as troubled about his gay identity as Hunky appeared to be. However, Mr. Shimata struggled more with his status as HIV+ in the workplace than any other interviewee I spoke with. Mr. Shimata was diagnosed prior to the advent of HAART and he felt he needed to disclose to people at work because he thought he might die and therefore needed to "give notice"; yet he was also diagnosed after the advent of AZT, the first pharmaceutical to treat HIV, so he knew there was treatment that might save him.

The thing that puts me off the most about talking about HIV in hospitals in Japan is that the first thing they ask you is how you got it. So you have to tell them about your sexuality. There are a lot of gay people who are out on TV and stuff, but actually, they are kind of special people. And in everyday life, everyday people don't really talk about their sexuality or their HIV status. Not at work, not at night [with partners]. Everyday people's knowledge about HIV is from like twenty years ago. Maybe the discrimination isn't so strong, but they still see it as a scary illness. So people can't be open about it. . . .

It took about a year to build up enough knowledge to be able to tell people in my life about my HIV status in a helpful way. In the beginning it was really hard because I didn't know much myself, and there were lots of times where there were misunderstandings. And I had to continue working so I had to control my health. . . .

I told the people in my section at work that I was HIV+ three months after my diagnosis. That caused a big panic. It's because I myself didn't have much knowledge or information about HIV. It became something to laugh about later, but they were shocked, and some people asked me repeatedly, "Are you going to die? When?" Even after three years, people would ask me if I was really OK. That's how it was . . . and that is how it still is for the general public [if you have HIV, you die]. . . . I started taking medicine two or three years later. Of course I was still living then, and all the people around me had thought I'd just die. But I didn't die after three years. Or five years. So they thought I was lying! I was healthy and working fine, so some of them were sure it was a lie. . . . So if you get cancer or something, you are often told, "you're going to die in six months" or three months, or whatever. So you have to tell your office [so I thought HIV was the same]. At the time, I thought I had a deadly disease, that I'd die, so I had to tell them. But, of course, I didn't. Now I think back and I probably didn't have to tell them anything at all. But, I didn't know. Now we have medicine, so there isn't that worry. . . .

I worked there for twenty years. Actually, it was a pretty good environment. The worst thing was that, at the time, there were a lot of people who were fired when their companies found out they had HIV. But in my case, even though it caused a huge panic in my office at first, I was able to explain about HIV to my co-workers as I learned myself . . . and because I did that, it prevented the panic from continuing. . . . So over time, they were able to understand. After a while, they stopped thinking about my HIV status . . . they stopped worrying about it . . . so now I tell people who have just found out to wait a little while before telling the people around them. They need to have a clear understanding [of the disease and its effects] before they tell other people. I mean, some people you can probably tell early on. But it depends on the person [you want to tell]. I tell them they should wait from six months to a year, until they have enough knowledge and information and have become able to talk about their status clearly, before telling most people. If you have to take leave to get medicine or care, it's OK to lie to your company, tell them it's another illness, until you're ready. . . .

Having HIV is only one part of you. Being gay is only one part of you. Your work is a part of you. There is no need, then, to focus on things like that completely . . . and it isn't necessary to tell everyone. . . . Someone at the hospital said, "You don't tell people at work you have athlete's foot, do you?" I was so surprised—this was twenty years ago when everyone was panicked and HIV meant you were going to die. But he was comparing it to athlete's foot! . . . Anyway, I realized it's not important to tell everyone, and "hiding" my status isn't necessarily a bad thing. As he said, it's only a part of me. (Mr. Shimata, 61, retired accountant)

Mr. Shimata's ability to access treatment, to learn about HIV and medications for it, and to translate what he learned to his coworkers enabled him to continue working despite his HIV status. Mr. Shimata was also the only interviewee who talked about the necessity of self-care *so that* he could work: in another conversation, he described making his own food and learning what foods were compatible with his ARVs. Ironically, his successful self-care made his coworkers question his status even more: they assumed—like he had initially—that he would get sick and die. When he didn't, they thought he was lying. Mr. Shimata then found himself in the position of having to reaffirm his status over and over until his coworkers came to terms with his diagnosis. This acceptance was facilitated by the fact that he was a good worker and that his team would suffer without his contributions. Given these experiences, it is perhaps not surprising that when asked about health, Mr. Shimata spent a lot of time describing his work situation, and how his experiences disclosing to his coworkers led him to conclude that *yōseisha* should take their time with disclosure and that it is better for their health if they disclose to people only after they have some measure of acceptance and understanding themselves. Taking the time to accept HIV as only a part of oneself is critical to mental and physical health.

Mr. Shimata was able to avoid questions from his family about his sexuality because he lives in a different region than they do, and he is the younger of several siblings, so the pressure to get married and have children has been alleviated by the childbearing of older, married siblings. What Hunky asserted about living in the Tokyo region versus the Osaka region held true in this case: Mr. Shimata could be somewhat "free" with regard to family responsibilities and maintaining privacy about his sexual orientation. Mr. Shimata's struggles to fulfill societal expectations of normative masculinity were mostly expressed through his focus on his workplace and the challenges of Japanese society's perceptions of HIV/AIDS.

Hunky and Mr. Shimata seem to have been able to sidestep societal expectations about reproduction through marital status and partner care, respectively; workplace contributions may have, over time, counteracted assumptions about perceived inability to work due to HIV status. As is evident from Mr. Shimata's case, sexuality was only really a concern if it resulted in illness and death, which would result in lost labor. But in the next case, the perceived threat to the body politic is much more direct.

HETEROSEXUAL INFECTION AND HAART: TAIYO

Taiyo is a heterosexual health professional who learned of his HIV status in 2010 at age 34. At the time of the interview, he had known his HIV status for less than a year. Demographically, he is most similar to Mr. Kawada: he is in his 30s and is heterosexual. But in terms of disease trajectory, he is actually more similar to Mr. Tamura and Mr. Shimata: he almost died from AIDS, even though he became infected with HIV long after HAART was developed. Although it was common to diagnose patients first with AIDS in the 1980s and early 1990s, most cases were caught earlier starting in mid-1990s. But cases like Taiyo's—where it does not occur to someone to get tested for HIV until they are showing symptoms of AIDS—are becoming more common. The Japanese medical community has started calling this trend, *ikinari eizu*—"suddenly, AIDS." It scares them because cases like Taiyo's seem to provide an example of HIV transmission despite years of (inadequate) sex education (Monobe et al. 2006), a focus on condoms for pregnancy prevention and not disease prevention[13] (Ikegami 2010), and/or the belief that HIV is a foreign problem, a sex work problem, or a problem among sexual minorities. Taiyo's HIV status scares the general public because Taiyo represents part of the public who are viewed as 'normal' and are assumed to contribute to Japanese society both in terms of labor and reproduction.

> When an internal medicine doctor first diagnosed me, he introduced me to a specialist in the same hospital. That specialist was an authority on HIV and had been to San Francisco and everything. He actually said, "Oh, you must be gay. You must like men," even though I didn't say anything about that. . . . He's actually a really good doctor and now I know he didn't mean it to be discriminatory like that, but I had a really bad first impression of him because of how he talked about these delicate issues.

> HIV is a problem in Japan, especially because people don't have correct knowledge about it. They don't really learn much about it in elementary or junior high schools. I myself don't remember when I first learned about HIV/AIDS. It's kind of embarrassing, but before I got it, I had no interest in HIV. I didn't have much awareness about it at all. My image was that it was this terrible illness. Now I know HIV is a strong illness, you can feel it physically. . . . Even though I have HIV, I think I'm healthy. I'm physically and mentally stable, and my life isn't much different than before. I enjoy it. Even though I'm not working now, I'll return to work soon, so I think I'm pretty healthy. . . . Taking care of your body, being able to work, and having motivation are all important parts of staying healthy. Because I was a nurse, I've been thinking about health for a while.
>
> Before [HIV] I used to hate comedy shows, but I had a "U-turn" after my diagnosis. I watched those shows and then I started making jokes. I gained my immunity back through laughter! In general, staying connected is important for yōseisha. We need to have people to talk to, people to share information with. I was hospitalized for two months, and then six months. Going home was hard because I lived alone. So having someone to talk to is really important. (Taiyo, age 35, nurse. October 9, 2011)

Like Mr. Kawada and Hunky, I met Taiyo at an HIV/AIDS event. Taiyo and Hunky were speakers who opted to explain their daily lives to the general public as a way for the public to learn about HIV (see Runestad 2016). In some ways, Taiyo is different from other *yōseisha* I met. He is the youngest *yōseisha* I interviewed, had known about his status for the shortest time, and did not identify as gay or as someone who had sex with other men. He was also trained as a nurse and was diagnosed with AIDS after developing lymphatic and intestinal cancers. After taking chemotherapy for the cancers and starting ART for HIV/AIDS, he was able to defeat cancer and is no longer living with AIDS. Like Mr. Tamura, Taiyo made a miraculous, Lazarus-like recovery. During a talk in the fall of 2011, he stated that his doctors predicted he would be dead before the event. He countered this with a defiant smile at the end of the talk, saying loudly, "But I'm still here!" When I met him again at an HIV/AIDS walk the following year, he looked fit and happy as he walked arm in arm with a female companion. Indeed, at the time of writing, Taiyo is still thriving.

Despite being trained as a nurse, Taiyo's prediagnosis understanding of HIV/AIDS and his definitions of health were in line with other *yōseisha*. Taiyo did not have a strong understanding of HIV and he was scared of the "terrible illness" when diagnosed. He thought he was going to die, and his physicians thought he was going to die, too. But his experiences as a nurse helped him believe in medications like chemotherapy for cancer and ARVs for HIV. Like Mr. Kawada, he notes the importance of self-care, and the relationship between mental and physical health: while in the hospital, he found that laughter and social connections were also central to his ability to regain his health.

Challenging assumptions about his sexuality and mode of infection caused him stress; however, at another event, I watched as he became visibly uncomfortable when audience members asked pointed questions about "promiscuity" in his life. It was clear that some audience members, when they could not assure themselves that the speaker's infection was caused by homosexual behaviors, attempted to allay their own fears by looking for another form of "deviance" that would explain Taiyo's infection and protect their own sense of safety. Having lived with HIV for less than a year at this point, it was harder for Taiyo than for other speakers to reframe the questions, focus on issues like condom use, and put the responsibility for protection back on the audience, which was often done by moderators or more experienced public *yōseisha* (Runestad 2016).

Taiyo's mode of transmission[14] and his heterosexual orientation resulted in greater stigma and discrimination compared to *yōseisha* like Mr. Kawada and Mr. Tamura who were infected iatrogenically. Although he is not gay and does not have to grapple with discrimination due to his sexuality like Hunky and Mr. Shimata, he does face challenges to his sexuality. Audience members probed him for past "bad" behavior connected to his HIV status and pushed for information about his current sex life. Clearly, they wanted to be able to reassure themselves of their own safety, while also wanting to place responsibility on him—and not themselves—for safe sex and breaking the transmission chain. In their eyes, Taiyo could be blamed (like Hunky and Mr. Shimata), and it was the responsibility of *yōseisha* to protect the Japanese body politic by policing their own sexual behaviors.

Despite these experiences, Taiyo returned to describing the ability to work as an important measure of his health and looked forward to returning to his job after these types of engagements. "I think I'm healthy . . . and my life isn't that different from before." He also explained that he also liked himself now better than he did before. He was uncertain then if he wanted a regular partner let alone a spouse and/or children, but he was well aware of the medical technologies available to him should he choose that path. Cullinane has documented the fear and discrimination HIV+ Japanese women have faced when they opt for marriage and children (2007). Further research is needed to determine whether Japanese society has become more accepting of these women in general, and how experiences of HIV+ men and women in serodiscordant partnerships differ.

CONCLUSION

Core aspects of being a "good Japanese" include being healthy so that one can contribute to society through work and reproduction. Going to college, getting a job, getting married, and having children are all signs that one is becoming a *shakaijin* and securing the future of Japan as a competitive nation-state on the global stage. As these five narratives demonstrate, an HIV diagnosis complicates these paths. Sometimes the complications are related to what the virus does to bodies, but more often in resource-rich Japan the complications come from perceptions about what being HIV+ does to social obligations. And sometimes those complications are more about prejudices regarding what it means to be a "normal" Japanese in the first place.

All five *yōseisha* highlighted here have shown that they have, to varying degrees, internalized sociocultural expectations about being a "good Japanese"—and sometimes this includes self-blame and stigma regarding their sexual identities or HIV status. All five men have, despite the ravages of HIV and other illnesses (ranging from cancer to hepatitis C and hemophilia), contributed to the workforce in jobs ranging from city worker to nurse to engineer. Mr. Kawada and Hunky are both happily married, although they describe the benefits of marriage in vastly different ways. Mr. Tamura and Mr. Shimata work as caregivers at home; Taiyo is a professional caregiver. It would be difficult to say that they are not contributing to Japanese society in terms of labor; if the frame is shifted from childbearing and filial piety to caring for others, it would be equally difficult to say that they are not benefitting Japanese society in terms of social support.

These men also have experienced different waves of HIV, different treatments and care responses, and differing access to resources based on the particulars of where they reside. They have different transmission routes and different responses to their roles in stopping the spread of HIV. Mr. Tamura, who contracted HIV iatrogenically, opted out of long-term sexual partnerships. Several years Mr. Tamura's junior, Taiyo continues to have an active sex life. But what becomes obvious in engaging in their narratives is how much they do to try to educate the general population about HIV, and how much the typical Japanese audience wants to be assured that they (the audience) are safe and fine—that they do not have to change their sexual behaviors because HIV is "over" in terms of *yakugai* transmission, or a problem of sexual minorities or a public health crisis in foreign countries and not in Japan. But the reality that *yakugai* cases are actual Japanese people—many of whom are still alive—is driven home by the presence of Mr. Kawada. The possibility of getting HIV as a heterosexual person is made clear by Taiyo's public appearances. And Mr. Shimata told me that he often tells audiences he was once one of them—an HIV+ Japanese person. And now, "I don't have HIV written on my forehead, but I'm right here."

Grappling with HIV has always been difficult, not just individually as described here but as a society as well. From learning about the virus and developing treatments, to building plans for treatment and prevention in various settings around the world, to considering how people age with it or experience syndemics—complications are everywhere. A further complication is that of cultural change. While the men presented in this chapter strived to be *shakaijin* in some ways, those ideals are also in constant flux and people from the same cultural background and generation may live them out in different ways. What it means to be a good person is redefined, sometimes in spite of challenges like HIV and sometimes because of it. We can see from these glimpses into engagements with HIV and Japanese identity that even in the places assumed to be homogenous and wealthy, no one's experiences of HIV are the same. And in those differences, perhaps we can see the seeds for broader understandings of what it means to live positively with HIV.

NOTES

1. I would like to thank my interviewees, without whom we would remain in the dark about some of the subtleties of HIV experiences in Japan. Thanks also go to David Murray for organizing our AAA panel and being a supportive and astute editor, and to my fellow panelists for their thoughtful comments.

2. *Yōseisha* literally means "positive person" and is used to describe someone who is HIV+. *Yōseisha* may or may not have progressed to AIDS.

3. There are other religious frameworks that have not had the same level of influence, such as Christianity (2% of the population), Ainu cosmology, the eclectic combinations of Buddhism and Shintoism found in the practices of mountain ascetics (*yamabushi*) and shamanesses (*itako*), fox possession, and "new" and "new-new" religious movements. For more on these, see Smyers (1999), Reader (1991), and Dubreuil and Fitzhugh (2001).

4. A less literal translation is "a life according to social expectations; a moral life."

5. For a full discussion of Japanese eugenics (from the late nineteenth century to 1945), see the work of Jennifer Robertson (2002), who argues that positive eugenics (family planning, safe birth initiatives, and theories of which sexual pairings would further the "Japanese race") and negative eugenics (sterilization of "undesirables") were both supported prior to World War II as a means of fostering a Japanese "race" that could stand up to foreign challenges.

6. The Japanese health insurance system codifies "levels of disability" as a means to allocate financial support, which is also likely to perpetuate the problematic associations between "disability," "poor health," and financial dependence rather than contributions.

7. Mother-to-child HIV infection is extremely low in Japan as all pregnant women are tested for HIV. However, 40% of Japan's hemophiliac population was infected with HIV through the use of tainted blood products imported from the United States prior to 1988 (see Seki et al. 2002).

8. Sex is the primary route of HIV infection in Japan, as access to injectable drugs is more restricted than in other countries, but drug use is increasingly becoming an issue there (see DiStefano 2016).

9. The National Diet is the formal name of the Legislature. Kawada is an elected official at the federal level.

10. The Habataki Project is a social welfare organization that aims to assist HIV-positive hemophiliacs.

11. Literally, "correct rule lifestyle"; a moral life.

12. Several Japanese HIV activists have used spoken or written narratives of their experiences in order to educate the Japanese public about HIV (Runestad 2016).

13. Condom use among heterosexual couples is more common in Japan among regular partners than during transaction sex or casual sex. The rationale is that the regular partner is a cared for partner, one that deserves protection, while a casual partner (particularly from the male perspective) is purely for fun. See Sandberg in Alexy and Cook (2018) for a discussion of condom negotiation.

14. Taiyo never directly disclosed his transmission to me, but insinuated it was through sexual contact.

REFERENCES

Alexy, Allison. 2011. "The Door My Wife Closed: Houses, Families, and Divorce in Contemporary Japan." In *Home and Family in Japan: Continuity and Transformation,* edited by Richard Ronald and Allison Alexy, 236–253. New York: Routledge.

Alexy, Allison and Emma Cook, eds. 2019. *Intimate Japan: Ethnographies of Closeness and Conflict.* Honolulu: University of Hawai`i Press.

Allison, Anne. 1994. *Nightwork: Sexuality, Pleasure, and Corporate Masculinity in a Tokyo Hostess Club.* Chicago: University of Chicago Press.

Befu, Harumi. 2001. *Hegemony of Homogeneity: An Anthropological Analysis of "Nihonjinron."* Melbourne: Trans Pacific Press.

Borovoy, Amy Beth. 2005. *The Too-good Wife: Alcohol, Codependency, and the Politics of Nurturance in Postwar Japan.* Berkeley: University of California Press.

Coulmas, Florian. 2008. *Population Decline and Ageing in Japan: The Social Consequences.* London: Routledge.

Cullinane, Joanne. 2007. "The Domestication of AIDS: Stigma, Gender, and the Body Politic in Japan." *Medical Anthropology Quarterly* 26 (3): 255–292.

Dales, Laura and Beverly Anne Yamamoto. 2019. "Romantic and Sexual Intimacy Before and Beyond Marriage." In *Intimate Japan: Ethnographies of Closeness and*

Conflict, edited by Allison Alexy and Emma E. Cook, 79–90. Honolulu: University of Hawai`i Press.

Dasgupta, Romit. 2006. "Salarymen Doing Straight: Heterosexual Men and the Dynamics of Gender Conformity." In *Genders, Transgenders, and Sexualities in Japan,* edited by Mark J. McLelland, 168–182. London: Routledge.

DiStefano, Anthony S. 2016. "HIV's Syndemic Links with Mental Health, Substance use, and Violence in an Environment of Stigma and Disparities." *Qualitative Health Research* 26 (7): 877–894.

Dubreuil, Chisato O. and William W. Fitzhugh, editors. 2001. *Ainu: Spirit of a Northern People.* Washington, DC: Arctic Studies Center at the Smithsonian National Museum of Natural History.

Frühstück, Sabine. 2003. *Colonizing Sex: Sexology and Social Control in Modern Japan.* Berkeley: University of California Press.

Hansen, Wilburn. 2007. "Eye on Religion: Shinto and the Japanese Attitude Toward Healing." *Southern Medical Journal* 100 (1): 118–119.

Ikegami, Chizuko. 2010. Founder of Place Tokyo. Personal communication.

Leupp, Gary. 1995. *Male Colors: The Construction of Homosexuality in Tokugawa Japan (1603—1868).* Berkeley: University of California Press.

Maree, Claire. 2015. "Queer Women's Culture and History in Japan." In *Routledge Handbook of Sexuality Studies in East Asia,* edited by Mark McLelland and Vera Mackie, 230–243. New York: Routledge.

McLelland, Mark. 2000. *Male Homosexuality in Modern Japan: Cultural Myths and Social Realities.* Richmond: Curzon.

McLelland, Mark. 2005. *Queer Japan From the Pacific War to the Internet Age.* Lanham: Rowman and Littlefield.

McLelland, Mark and Vera Mackie, eds. 2015. *Routledge Handbook of Sexuality Studies in East Asia.* New York: Routledge.

Miller, Elizabeth. 2002. "What's in a Condom? HIV and Sexual Politics in Japan." *Culture, Medicine, and Psychiatry* 26 (1): 1–32.

Miller, Laura and Jan Bardsley. 2005. *Bad Girls of Japan.* Hampshire: Palgrave Macmillan.

Monobe, Hirofumi, Takuya Ishibashi, Yutaka Satoh, Jyun Fukuda, and Masahiro Yoda. 2006. "Shōgakkō ni okeru sei kyōiku no jirei kenkyu: HIV kansen yobō no tame ni Shōgakkō dankai ni okeru sei kyōiku [A Case Study of Sex Education in an Elementary School: Sex Education at the Elementary School Level for the Prevention of HIV]." Yokohama Kokuritsu Daigaku: 239–248.

Nakamura, Karen. 2013. *A Disability of the Soul: An Ethnography of Schizophrenia and Mental Illness in Contemporary Japan.* Ithaca: Cornell University Press.

National Institute of Infectious Diseases (NIID). 2017a. "HIV/AIDS in Japan, 2017." https://www.niid.go.jp/niid/en/iasr-vol38-e/865-iasr/8335-463te.html

NIID. 2017b. "Notifications of HIV cases and AIDS Patients in Japan by Top 10 Prefectures in 2017." https://www.niid.go.jp/niid/images/iasr/2018/09/463tet01.gif

NIID. 2017c. "Cumulative Reported Number of HIV Cases and AIDS Patients, 1985–2017, Japan." https://www.niid.go.jp/niid/images/iasr/2018/09/463tef01.gif

NIID. 2017d. "Annual reported Number of New HIV Cases and AIDS Patients, 1985–2017, Japan." https://www.niid.go.jp/niid/images/iasr/2018/09/463tef02.gif

NIID. 2017e. "Reported Number of New Japanese Male HIV Cases and AIDS Patients by Mode of Transmission, 1985–2017, Japan." https://www.niid.go.jp/niid/images/iasr/2018/09/463tef03.gif

NIID. 2017f. "Reported Number of New Japanese Male HIV Cases and AIDS Patients Due to Homosexual Contact By Age Group, 1985–2017." https://www.niid.go.jp/niid/images/iasr/2018/09/463tef04.gif

Pflugfelder, Gregory. 1999. *Cartographies of Desire: Male-male Sexuality in Japanese Discourse, 1600–1950.* Berkeley: University of California Press.

Reader, Ian. 1991. *Religion in Contemporary Japan.* Honolulu: University of Hawai`i Press.

Reader, Ian and George Tanabe. 1998. *Practically Religious: Worldly Benefits and the Common Religion of Japan.* Honolulu: University of Hawai`i Press.

Robertson, Jennifer. 2002. "Blood Talks: Eugenic Modernity and the Creation of the New Japanese." *History and Anthropology* 13 (3): 191–216.

Runestad, Pamela L. 2010. What People Think Matters: The Relationship between Perceptions and Epidemiology in the JAPANESE HIV Epidemic. *International Journal of Interdisciplinary Social Sciences*, 5 (4), 331–344.

Runestad, Pamela L. 2016. "Walking The Walk, Talking The Talk: Narratives that Challenge HIV/AIDS Taboos in Japan." *Asia Pacific Perspectives* 14 (1): 28–49.

Sawada, Janine. 2014. *Practical Pursuits: Religion, Politics and Personal Cultivation in Nineteenth-Century Japan.* Honolulu: University of Hawai`i Press.

Seki, Yukiko, Yoshihiko Yamazakai, Yoji Inoue, C Wakabayashi, and S. Seto. 2002. "How HIV Infected Haemophiliacs in Japan Were Informed of Their HIV-positive Status." *AIDS Care* 14 (5): 651–664.

Shigematsu, Setsu. 2015. "The Women's Liberation Movement and Sexuality in Japan." In *The Routledge Handbook of Sexuality Studies in East Asia,* edited by Mark McLelland and Vera Mackie, 174–187.

Smyers, Karen Ann. 1999. *The Fox and the Jewel: Shared and Private Meanings in Contemporary Japanese Inari Worship.* Honolulu: University of Hawai`i Press.

Stevens, Carolyn. 2007. "Living with Disability in Urban Japan." *Japanese Studies* 27 (3): 263–278.

Sugimoto, Yoshio. 2003. *An Introduction to Japanese Society.* Cambridge: Cambridge University Press.

Teruyama, Junko. 2014. "Japan's New Minority: Persons with Hattatsu Shogai (Developmental Disability)." PhD Diss, Department of Anthropology, University of Michigan.

Visscher, Cindy. 2006. "Eye on Religion: Understanding the Cultural/Religious Melange in Treating Japanese Patients." *Southern Medical Journal* 99 (12): 1448–1449.

Weiner, Michael. 1997. *Japan's Minorities: The Illusion of Homogeneity.* London: Routledge.

Chapter 7

Opting Out

Aging Gays, HIV/AIDS, and the Biopolitics of Queer Viral Time

David A. B. Murray

In[1] the midst of mostly optimistic headlines in North American newspapers with headlines like "End to AIDS in sight as huge study finds drugs stop HIV transmission" (Boseley and Devline 2019; see also McKinley 2019) and declarations from public health organizations that HIV/AIDS is now a manageable, chronic illness,[2] a group of older gay men who have been living with HIV for many decades gathers fortnightly in downtown Toronto to "deal with reality" as one member put it, and to "take things in our own hands." In this chapter, I want to focus on the ways in which members of this group discuss their everyday experiences, their relationships to various aspects of the HIV/AIDS apparatus, their observations of the past, present, and future, and their decision to "take things in our own hands" in order to better understand the disjunctive biopolitics of what I call queer viral time.

In mainstream "end of crisis" discourses, the narrative arc of HIV/AIDS has shifted from one of tragedy, suffering, and death to one of hope, optimism, and life, primarily in relation to the widespread success of antiretroviral therapy (ART) drug regimens since the late 1990s, which have resulted in a substantial global drop in deaths from AIDS, albeit with substantially different rates for different regions and/or key populations (see Introduction to this book). As a result, in many parts of the world, HIV infection is now referred to as a "chronic" rather than "terminal" disease, such that many people living with HIV are now told they will not die from AIDS-related complications as long as they adhere to an ART regimen. This profound change in the biomedical status of a disease, along with recent biomedical discoveries such as the Undetectable=Untransmissable (U=U) campaign, based on the knowledge that a person who is on ART and has an undetectable viral load cannot transmit the virus to anyone, conveys a message that the crisis is over for those people living with HIV (PLHIV) as they can live "near normal" lifespans and everyday lives. However, as numerous HIV/AIDS researchers and activists have pointed out, "the end of the AIDS crisis" and "AIDS as a chronic illness" narratives are highly contested and carry within them problematic biomedical assumptions about time, health, personhood, and sociality that do not engage with the fluidity and flexibility of disease conditions over the life course (Colvin 2011, Manderson and Smith Morris 2010, Sangaramoorthy 2018), and do not question where, how, why, and for whom AIDS may or may not be ending (Benton, Sangaramoorthy and Kalofonos 2017, 474). In other words, "Treatment narratives that celebrate HIV's long-awaited arrival as a chronic condition mask the persistence of the local and global structural conditions that produced vulnerability and infection in the past and continued suffering and poor therapeutic adherence in the present" (Colvin 2011). Those whose course of illness doesn't fit the biomedically defined model of a stable and manageable chronic illness may come to be viewed in their communities and health systems as defaulters, failed subjects, or unfortunate statistical outliers (Colvin 2011, Mattes 2014).

Thus, if we acknowledge that HIV as "chronic illness" should be recognized as a status that is fluid and flexible and may have differing impacts on differentially positioned social groups, and that biotechnical interventions may address and control some of the physiological symptoms of HIV as chronic illness, but not necessarily the psychological or social ones, "then the chronicity of an illness experience is not (only) a medical fact but (also) a technological, political and economic one" (Smith Morris in Sangaramoorthy 2018). Based on this interpretation of chronic illness, Sangaramoorthy proposes "a reorientation of (the) logic of (HIV) chronicity to one that regards HIV as a continual crisis as it is lived and experienced for many around the world" (2018, 3).

In this chapter, the comments and conversations of a group of older, gay, white men in Toronto, all of whom have been living with HIV for more than 20 years, support this reoriented logic of HIV chronicity. For them, the crisis is not over despite the advent of ART and more recent biomedical findings such as U=U. As will be outlined in greater detail below, members of this group encounter ongoing and new challenges in their day-to-day lives reflecting a particular intersection of biomedical (HIV+), sociosexual (gay), age (over 55), racial (white), economic (limited income), and gender (cis-men) statuses and experiences. These challenges include (1) physical afflictions and ailments associated with aging bodies, prior AIDS-related illnesses, and/or decades of ingesting toxic HIV medications; (2) navigating a complex bureaucratic public health care system in order to adequately address multiple health concerns; (3) dealing with HIV/AIDS service organizations' (HASOs) increasingly professionalized and bureaucratic cultures; (4) accessing appropriate support in Toronto HASOs that are adapting programs and services to the increasing ethno-racial, age, migrant, and socioeconomic diversity of the PLHIV population in the greater Toronto area; and (5) their own (gay) community's HIV/AIDS amnesia, and its increasingly uncritical acceptance of biomedical knowledge as undisputable fact.

I argue that these challenges, arising from the intersection of viral, sexual orientation, gender, income, age, and race statuses, disrupt notions of time embedded in hegemonic biomedical definitions of HIV as a chronic illness: They produce a perception of being out of time, or put slightly differently, these older, gay, white, HIV+ men's orientations, memories, experiences, and perceptions produce a particular form of *queer viral time* that is "out of joint" with official chronologies and definitions of HIV/AIDS, which form part of what I call *homonormative time*, where the shift from a terminal to chronic status of being HIV+ is framed through a return to normality and inclusivity, and as part of an inevitable movement toward the end of the AIDS crisis for LGBTQ communities. I argue that queer viral time, a disease-based time out of joint, is anachronic in relation to homonormative temporal arcs of "HIV as chronic disease" narratives, as it reveals a perceptual discrepancy between how members of this group sense their place in the world around them and the way in which they feel they are placed in (or erased from) contemporary HIV/AIDS and mainstream LGBTQ narratives about the past, present, and future. This sense of shared anachrony is simultaneously liberating, alienating, and infuriating for members of this group, and helps to illustrate the importance of paying attention to the temporal dynamics of complex subject formations defined through/by chronic illness in order to better understand the social, political, and economic dimensions of biomedical health discourses and their effects.

Queer viral time, an anachronic orientation toward hegemonic HIV/AIDS chronicity and end of crisis narratives, also contributes to a better understanding of the biopolitics of HIV/AIDS, that is, a political economy of life defined through disease management which aims to administer, secure, develop, and foster the lives of those living with HIV. This group's anachronic position in relation to contemporary HIV/AIDS discourses reveals both the power of and resistance to these discourses and their development through disciplines such as statistics, demography, and epidemiology, which attempt to govern HIV+ individuals and groups by practices of correction, exclusion, normalization, disciplining, therapeutics, and optimization (Lemke 2010, 429–430). These men's critiques of "end of HIV/AIDS crisis" narratives, new prevention and treatment regimes that rely entirely on pharmaceutical interventions (such as U=U or PrEP[3]), and overly bureaucratic HASOs push back against contemporary forms of HIV/AIDS governance and are generated through long-term memories and experiences of pain and loss, as well as skepticism borne from battling indifferent medical and government institutions through the first decades of the pandemic. Their memories and experiences, which are integral to the formation of queer viral time, also draw attention to the temporal dimensions of biopolitical processes: If an analytics of biopolitics is based on investigating "the network of relations between power strategies, knowledge practices and modes of subjectivation" (Lemke 2010, 432), then that analytics must also factor in how power strategies, knowledge practices, and modes of subjectivation employ particular arrangements of, or assumptions about, time that contribute toward definitions of optimal or normalized subjects.

At the same time, this group's critique of local HASOs prioritizing the needs of "other" PLHIV populations ("other" being defined through age, gender, ethnicity, race, migrant status, or heterosexual orientation) reveals a particular orientation toward the contemporary demographic reality of PLHIV in Toronto reflecting the racial, age, sociosexual and gender homogeneity and insularity of the group, and discriminatory attitudes that emanate from such homogeneity, which in turn reveals some of the sociopolitical tensions and inequities within PLHIV communities and HASOs in large urban contexts.

Finally, I will argue that the anachronic disposition of this group challenges the frameworks of much research on HIV/AIDS and aging: While federal and international health organizations now acknowledge the distinct needs of "an aging HIV+ population" (Government of Canada 2016, UNAIDS 2013), this population remains vaguely defined and understudied: most Canadian HIV/AIDS data has just one category for older adults ("50+"), likely an artifact of the "pretreatment" era when few people with HIV survived past a certain age (Leahy 2017). In 2020, gay and queer men who were diagnosed with HIV 20 or more years ago could span in age range from their late 30s to 70s and beyond, but discussions about HIV among this group have mostly focused on biomedical concerns for aging (50+) bodies, such as higher rates of multiple chronic conditions (UNAIDS 2013, 2016). While some researchers and HIV/AIDS organizations have also noted psychosocial issues for aging PLHIV such as isolation, stigma, and depression (CATIE 2010, 2016, Ontario HIV Treatment Network 2012, McDonald et al. 2013), there appears to be little research that applies intersectional, critical temporal, and reflexive analytical frameworks to PLHIV experiences of living and aging with the virus for a significant portion of their lifespans.

The research findings in this chapter are from an ethnographic research project focusing on how differentially positioned PLHIV and organizations servicing PLHIV populations in Toronto are navigating "end of the HIV/AIDS crisis" discourses, the circulation of new biomedical knowledge about HIV (such as PrEP and U=U campaigns), and daily challenges of living with

HIV in a period of decreasing funding for and public interest in HIV/AIDS. Over a period of 15 months in 2018–2019, I volunteered at two Toronto HASOs and participated in four support groups for PLHIV in order to learn how therapeutic interventions for PLHIV are designed and implemented, as well as to observe how differentially positioned PLHIV (dis)engage with these programs. Three of these groups were organized by HASOs or hospitals with HIV research units, but the group discussed in this chapter was purposefully independent of any existing HASOs and had no institutional affiliation.

My HIV status facilitated entry into most of the groups as they were limited to PLHIV. I was motivated to join in part out of personal interest to find more accurate information that might be helpful in addressing my own curiosity and anxieties about aging and HIV—I was reading different and often conflicting reports about the impact of long-term infection and a lifetime of antiretroviral medications, increased comorbidities, and mental health issues—and in part out of professional anthropological interest to see how social differences and inequities informed counseling and support for differentially positioned PLHIV in Toronto. In addition, my white, cisgender, queer-identified, and long-term PLHIV status facilitated admission to the group that I focus on in this chapter, as it was restricted to gay men who had been living with HIV for many years. I informed the group facilitator that I was participating as both as a PLHIV and a researcher, and was granted access as long as I introduced myself to the group as both a "valid" member (an older gay man who had been living with HIV for many years) and researcher, and agreed to follow all group norms, which included guaranteeing the confidentiality and anonymity of all group members.

After a brief description of the group's formation, structure, and membership below, I will then present some excerpts from group meetings' conversations in order to convey these men's experiences with the individuals, bureaucracies, and organizations that form part of the HIV/AIDS apparatus in Toronto, which will help to illustrate the anachronic orientation of queer viral time and the complicated affects that result from it.

LIVING LIKE LAZARUS

I learned about this group's existence while interviewing a former director of a nonprofit organization dedicated to supporting individuals and families impacted by HIV/AIDS. She put me in touch with Thomas, the group facilitator, who then wanted to meet me prior to a group meeting in order to explain the group's objectives and interests and to confirm that I met the basic criteria for group admission. Before our meeting, Thomas informed me in a text message that the group is only for gay identified men who have been living with HIV for a prolonged period of time (this period was not defined, although as I would soon discover, most members have been HIV+ for more than 20 years). At our first meeting at a restaurant in the core of Toronto's "gay village," Thomas, who looked to be in his early 60s, greeted me with a friendly smile and began by telling me that the group was totally separate from any other (HIV/AIDS service) organization in Toronto: "We have issues with them . . . so we're doing things for ourselves." He then handed me a photocopied set of notes that described the group's formation and its principles: The group had been going for about 15 years and was formed through a network of gay men living with HIV in and around Toronto who had stopped attending local HASOs for various reasons (some of which will be outlined below). Thomas explained to me that this group of gay men was dealing with the challenge of being alive after they had believed for many years that they would die from AIDS, because they were diagnosed before the systematic rollout of ART. The photocopied notes referred to this as the "Lazarus Syndrome," a term found in some HIV/AIDS literature to describe how individuals suffering from AIDS symptoms and often near death were "saved" by the arrival of ART treatment and thus "raised from the dead." Thomas added that the group was also formed out of their shared sense that no existing HASO was adequately addressing issues that matter to them. He went on to tell me that the group had no leaders and no particular format. Rather, at each meeting, members talked about their experiences, and particular themes would then organically emerge. Thomas repeatedly pointed out that this was not a "therapy or support" group like those found in some of the HASOs, where there were particular agendas and/or therapeutic objectives.

Once Thomas confirmed that I met the minimum criteria for group membership and understood their purpose and guidelines, I was invited to attend the meetings, which took place every two weeks in the meeting room of a LGBTQ friendly organization located in downtown Toronto.[4] Over the six months of meetings that I attended, attendance ranged from five to eight members with a couple of new members joining over that period of time. All of the group members identified as gay men who had been living with HIV for 20 to 30 (or more) years, ranged in age from 50s to mid-70s, and appeared to be white/Caucasian.[5] At least half of the members lived in Toronto public housing units and had received income support through the Ontario Disability Service Program for many years as they could not work due to HIV-related health issues (some were now receiving Canada Pension Plan payments). The majority had been members of the group for five years or longer, and most group members had known each other for many years. Some were clearly friends outside the group (they would mention social events with each other during group conversations), while others did not appear to socialize with anyone from the group. Thomas told me that the group did not have any online presence, and that membership, for the most part, was based on word-of-mouth recruitment, that is, through group members inviting people they knew to join the group. This form of recruitment may help to explain the group's relatively homogenous sexual orientation, age, race, and long-term HIV-status composition.

GOING BACKWARD

Each meeting would begin with a couple of minutes of silence in order to remember those who had lost their lives to AIDS. This would be followed by a check-in where each group member would talk about how things were going since the last meeting and/or raise issues they would like to be discussed at the present or future meetings. Most members' check-ins would include a brief summary or update of their health status, as many had multiple ailments and conditions that required regular visits to doctors' offices or specialists in hospitals. At the check-in of a late summer 2018 meeting, Rod, a long-term member of the group, recounted how the previous week he had driven from his home to St. Michael's hospital in downtown Toronto to get an MRI (magnetic resonance imaging) scan for a neuromuscular disease, but on the way back home he had a car accident, which he thought was due to having taken Ativan, an antianxiety medication, to deal with his anxiety of hospitals. Luckily, no one was injured, but as a result, Rod's license was suspended, due to his chronic neuromuscular medical condition which ostensibly rendered him unsafe to drive. Rod was angry, because he was sure the accident was due to being drowsy from too much Ativan (a one-time occurrence, he maintained), not his neuromuscular disease. Now he would have to take Wheel-Trans, the Toronto public transit system for people with disabilities, to do all his errands, which would be time consuming and frustrating. Furthermore, he wouldn't be able to drive out of town to help an old friend who was dying from cancer, and he was worried about how his friend would cope.

Rod's predicament generated a lively discussion among the group members, some recounting similar feelings of anxiety when visiting hospitals and similar problems with perceived misdiagnoses. Robert, another long-term member, told Rod he understood these feelings of anxiety and resentment when visiting hospitals: A few weeks ago, he had gone to see a dermatologist at a downtown hospital for skin cancer treatment. When the doctor entered the room, he read Robert's chart, looked at him, and said "Aren't you people all dead?" Whether or not the question was meant as a joke, Robert was shocked, and didn't know how to respond, so he just sat there looking down at the floor. Ben, another member whose facial features displayed the effects of lipodystrophy (a loss of fat in the cheekbones), was told by a doctor at a local clinic to make his next appointment at the downtown hospital where the doctor also worked, because he was "scaring the patients" at the clinic. After a few other similar anecdotes, Thomas, the facilitator, said, "it feels like we're going backwards" when it comes to how group members were being treated in doctors' offices and hospitals, and "that's why we need to be here (at the group meetings) in order to give each other support." The group also discussed the importance of being "selectively honest" with their doctors and/or government officials, so that they would not lose resources, freedoms, and/or access to financial support. The feeling of going backward and the need for strategic engagement with the public health apparatus were oft-repeated remarks that would emerge in relation to a variety of conversation topics.

ALIENATION IN HASOS

Another common conversational topic revolved around members' encounters with local HASOs. When Thomas learned that I was volunteering at one organization providing support services for people living with HIV/AIDS, he told me why he has "nothing to do with them anymore": A few years ago, he had gone there to request some help to cover the cost of a pair of glasses, which he couldn't afford as he was living on disability benefits. One of the programs of this organization provided financial assistance to its clients for health-related costs, so Thomas thought his request for glasses would be accepted. He met with a social worker at the organization who said this would not be a problem, just provide them with a prescription and receipt for the glasses, and a check would be ready in a few weeks. However, when Thomas returned a couple of weeks later, he was told by the person at the front reception desk that there was no check and that the cost of glasses was not eligible for reimbursement. Thomas was upset, and when he asked why no one had contacted him about this decision, he was told that an email had been sent to him. "But the social worker knew I didn't have a computer, so I just flipped out. When a manager came out and asked 'what's the problem,' I said I am not happy with treatment here, I'm not getting any help, so you'll never hear from me again." Other members recounted similar stories of problematic encounters with this and other HASOs. Rod said that if you find out you're HIV+ and go to (another large HASO), "they put you in a group for 10 weeks and then let you go." Ben said he used to volunteer with that organization, but now it's "all about a degree" (referring to the professional credentials of staff members) and it has become "too much of a bureaucracy." The discussion ended with members nodding their heads in agreement when Thomas summed up the general consensus of the group by saying "all of us (have) stopped going to the HASOs . . . there is no place to turn to . . . (except) here . . . where we can get advice from each other and find the right people to talk to."

In these conversations, feelings of frustration and disenchantment with the HASOs reflected a sense of marginalization and alienation from the very organizations that were created by and for these men in the 1980s and 1990s. However, in subsequent decades, members of the group observed changes to the structure and programs of these HASOs: They have become increasingly bureaucratized through gradual enmeshment in the state-funded public health system, and they are increasingly staffed by employees with specialized training and education such as social work, psychology, or nursing.[6] This sense of marginalization and alienation reflected a sense of being "out of place" in the very places which they were once a central part of.

PREP AND BIG PHARMA

One other topic that emerged more than once in group meetings and elicited spirited conversation was PrEP, an HIV prevention strategy where HIV-negative individuals take anti-HIV medications before coming into contact with HIV to reduce their risk of becoming infected. During the period in which I attended meetings, PrEP occupied center stage as a new HIV prevention strategy in Toronto and was much discussed in LGBTQ media as well as promoted heavily by some local HASOs, Canadian HIV/AIDS organizations, and local and federal public health services.[7] At one group meeting, where the conversation had turned to frustrations with some Toronto HASOs, Thomas mentioned one of the reasons he was frustrated:

> (The HASO) is too obsessed with PrEP. The drug companies are paying them huge sums, and for people there it's all about keeping (their) jobs. Nobody talks about how these drugs have side effects, nobody knows what the effects of PrEP will be ten years down the road. . . . The pitch for PrEP is just like the pitch for AZT.[8] . . . Trust me, we've seen what the meds can do . . . they all have side effects. There is no pill to erase AIDS![9]

At another meeting, PrEP was mentioned again when members discussed the recent Toronto LGBTQ Pride Parade (June 2018): One member stated that the parade was full of pharmaceutical companies and their floats for PrEP and ART drugs, which mostly consisted of good-looking men carrying placards along the parade route or cute gay couples staring out at the crowd on posters mounted on balloon-festooned flatbed trucks. Robert stated that PrEP now dominates all LGBTQ and HIV/AIDS events like the Pride Parade and World AIDS day (December 1) and that these "sales pitches" were "brainwashing" people: "AIDS day should be about AIDS, not PrEP."

The group's perspective on PrEP campaigns is highlighted through Thomas's comparison of PrEP to one of the first widely distributed AIDS medications, AZT, in the late 1980s and early 1990s, and his reminder that "we've seen what the meds can do."[10] The group's shared skepticism and distrust of a biomedical solution to help prevent the spread of HIV comes from these men's memories of their battles with governments and pharmaceutical companies to find, obtain, and/or finance treatment for HIV in the first decades of the epidemic, as well as their subsequent suffering with debilitating side effects from first wave HIV medications like AZT. Thomas's comments also implicitly convey the activism of previous generations of gay men living with and impacted by HIV/AIDS, such as the Toronto-based group AIDS Action Now, formed in 1988, which was dedicated to fighting government indifference and barriers to treatment. AIDS Action Now activities included sustained protests against and negotiations with provincial and federal governments and international pharmaceutical companies in order to facilitate rapid distribution of effective treatment protocols which resulted in accelerated and affordable access to effective medications for PLHIV (McCaskell 2006).

The group members' shared skepticism and frustration with contemporary Toronto HASOs' "obsession" with PrEP as a method to prevent HIV transmission (i.e., their unquestioning reliance on a biomedical intervention and ipso facto, the pharmaceutical industry), along with their invocation of AZT as a historical example to critique popular contemporary HIV discourses painting a picture of a rosy future on PrEP, illustrates the group's "out of joint" orientation toward the priorities and narratives of the HIV/AIDS organizations that they helped create, but who now appear to be the happy handmaidens of the governments and corporations they fought for decades. This out of joint temporal orientation can also be viewed as a biopolitical intervention, as it challenges the normative chronology inherent in HIV/AIDS knowledge production, in which new pharmaceutical treatments like PrEP are presented as evidence of inevitable progress toward the end of the HIV/AIDS crisis through biomedical interventions.

GRUMPY OLD (GAY WHITE) MEN?

After attending the first couple of group meetings, I thought that the timbre of conversations amounted to just another version of "Grumpy Old Men," the well-worn cliché (and 1993 Hollywood film) describing the general demeanor of a gendered generation defined by the passage of time. While this stereotype speaks volumes about the ways in which time, age, gender, and affect are interconnected in popular Euro-American age-based social identity constructs, I soon realized that it was inaccurate and unhelpful in reference to understanding this group of long-term HIV+ gay men's affective dispositions toward contemporary HIV/AIDS discourses, policies, and support services, as well as their own LGBTQ community. While irritability and dissatisfaction may be common affective components in any conversation about present-day realities evaluated through memories of the past, for this particular group these affects are the result of specific, shared memories and experiences based on viral infection at a specific point in epidemiological time; collective action in response to societal silence and fear around HIV; and shared gender, sexual, and racial orientations, which together form what I have called queer viral time.

Long-term living and aging in queer viral time produces a particular affective orientation through memories of suffering, solidarity, resistance, and endurance formed in an era of fear, trauma, and death, which is then applied to a present-day reality of relative silence, rejection, and/or marginalization in the very locations and communities that are supposed to provide assistance and support. Long-term living and aging in queer viral time is a variation on "queer time," which is built on critiques of heteronormative, reproductive, "future-oriented," and chronological frameworks of time (i.e., Edelson 2004, Halberstam 2005). Halberstam argues that "queer subcultures produce alternative temporalities by allowing their participants to believe that their futures can be imagined according to logics that lie outside of those paradigmatic markers of life experience—namely birth, marriage, reproduction and death" (2005:2). This group of long-term HIV+ gay men has indeed produced an alternative queer temporality, but one that is not shared by most other queer subcultures: They have lived into a future what was not supposed to happen and have seen their lives "resurrected" through the transformation of their health status from terminal to chronic through a sustained, friction-filled relationship with biomedical, pharmaceutical, and governmental apparatuses. They have witnessed profound transformations in public and institutional responses to the epidemic, from intense public scrutiny, panic, ignorance and fear, to complacency and now invisibility. Perhaps even more disturbing for them, this complacency and invisibility has occurred within their own LGBTQ community and many of its organizations.

Long-term living and aging in queer viral time is also a critique of what I have called homonormative time, a time that is defined through a linear chronological narrative of LGBTQ activism that ends in the present moment of inclusivity and equality, such that all Canadian LGBTQ citizens now ostensibly enjoy the same rights, responsibilities, and privileges as their heterosexual Canadian counterparts. Homonormative time now includes an optimistic future component in which HIV/AIDS, while still acknowledged as a concern for the community, is mostly framed as a problem that can be imminently contained and eliminated through biomedical interventions like U=U and PrEP. This homonormative present and future time is distinct from the group's queer viral time and produces a sense of alienation and frustration, or what I call time out of joint, for group members who are living in queer viral time.

Finally, long-term living and aging in queer viral time confirms and challenges the temporal assumptions of "AIDS generation" narratives, which claim that members of gay communities in the 1980s and 1990s share a collective identity formed through the trauma and activism of the first two decades of the AIDS pandemic and that survivors of this generation in the present-day manifest characteristics of resilience and strength (i.e., Halkitis 2013). While the support group members clearly have a similar perspective on contemporary HIV discourses and support services formed through a shared set of experiences demarcated by a particular point in time (being HIV+ in the first decades of the pandemic prior to the rollout of ART), their ongoing frustration with "end of crisis" HIV narratives, the public health care system, HASOs, and their own LGBTQ community, interrupts the homonormative chronological assumption of the AIDS generation belonging to a moment in the past that is no longer relevant and/or has subsequently been replaced by newer generational identities.[11]

However, we must also acknowledge that queer viral time has multiple instantiations produced through different intersections of experience and identification. In other words, there is no singular queer viral time—this group of older gay men who have lived with HIV for decades do not share the same experiences as a 25-year-old queer racialized nonbinary individual in Toronto who has just been diagnosed HIV+ in 2019, or a middle-aged cisgender heterosexual woman from Nigeria who has been living with HIV for a decade and recently migrated to Canada as a refugee. In the group meetings, there was occasional acknowledgment of and disidentification with other trajectories of viral time, reflecting the homogenous racial, sexual, age, and gender orientations and experiences of group members. For instance, in one of the group discussions about local HASOs and their apparent lack of interest in sustainably serving and supporting older HIV+ gay men, Ben noted how the demographics of HIV infection are changing in Toronto: "Gay men are still getting it, but there are more women, more people on drugs and more immigrants." Thomas made a similar comment at another meeting but added an evaluative element: "They (the HASO) prioritize people on the streets, intravenous drug users, refugees and immigrants . . . (they are) spreading (themselves) too thinly."

Ben and Thomas's observations on the changing demographics of PLHIV in Toronto are borne out by epidemiological data: In Toronto, over 20,000 people have been diagnosed with HIV in Toronto since 1985, and the AIDS Committee of Toronto (ACT) estimates that about 10,000 Torontonians are currently living with HIV (ACT 2018). Men continue to contract HIV at significantly higher rates than women, and of the males diagnosed with HIV in Toronto 2013, 79% were men who have sex with men (City of Toronto 2015). However, additional populations that continue to face a higher burden of HIV infection include injecting drug users; indigenous persons; African, Caribbean, and Black communities; and persons who come from areas of the world where HIV infection is more common (City of Toronto 2015, Government of Canada 2016). More recently, an Ontario HIV Epidemiology and Surveillance Initiative (OHESI) report on new HIV diagnoses in Ontario found that "between 2012 to 2017, there was an increase in the proportion of new HIV diagnoses where the individuals were Black males, East/Southeast Asian males, Arab/West Asian males, Latin American males and White females" (OHESI 2019). During my time volunteering in a Toronto HASO in 2017–2018, I heard comments from staff and clients that supported these statistics and the group members' observations: They noted how, over the past decade, there was a discernable change in who was "coming in through the front door" (i.e., less gay white men, and more heterosexual men and women, recently arrived migrants, visible minorities and/or people facing intersectional challenges like mental health and homelessness) and that support services and programs had to adapt to a wider range of challenges presented by this increasingly diverse PLHIV clientele.

However, Ben and Thomas's comments were not just neutral observations about demographic shifts in Toronto's HIV+ population: When they said HASOs are "prioritizing" other groups and "spreading too thinly" they were critiquing these organizations for not continuing to focus on their own needs and challenges, and they were conveying a sense of resentment spurred through their perception of being abandoned by the very organizations they (or their ilk) worked so hard to establish. This critique, borne out of a sense of abandonment, emanates from a particular version of queer viral time that began decades ago when HIV/AIDS in Toronto was an epidemic ravaging a group of cisgender white men who identified as "gay" and mostly socialized with other gay white men. Thus, this version of queer viral time has a particular chronology and conglomeration of affects (some discriminatory) that are defined in part through age, sexual, gender, and ethno-racial orientations.

My observation that queer viral time has racial, sexual, gendered, and age-based dimensions resonates with a long lineage of critical social science research identifying the socioeconomic and political dynamics of the pandemic: The intersectionality of HIV vulnerability with structural forms of inequality based on race, class, gender, and sexuality on multiple scales (local, national, and global) has been well documented in the HIV/AIDS research literature (see, e.g., Farmer 1999 and 2003, Hoad 2007, Jolivette 2016, Moyer 2015, Patton 2002, Sangaramoothy 2014, and Stockdill 2003). These group members' remarks therefore illustrate how PLHIV have differential relationships to intersecting forms of social inequality, such that in this case, the long-term racial, age, and sexual homogeneity of this group produce feelings of disidentification and resentment toward PLHIV of different backgrounds reflecting particular arrangements of privilege and marginalization.

CONCLUSION

At a historical moment when local, national, and international public health organizations are claiming that the end of the HIV/AIDS epidemic is near, the conversations of a small group of older, long-term HIV+, gay, white men in Toronto produce an astutely different narrative. In these conversations, memories of suffering and loss and activist responses to public indifference and state inaction during a time of crisis are applied to contemporary encounters with the public health care system, HASOs, and the LGBTQ community, often resulting in collective irritation and skepticism toward "end of crisis" discourses, new pharmaceutical interventions, and the HIV/AIDS apparatus in general. These men's comments disrupt the hegemonic biomedical narrative arc of the transformation of HIV's status from terminal to chronic, and HIV+ lives from imminent death to "near normal." Their shared experience of HIV's gradual shift from the center to the margins of public health concerns, as well as its gradual disappearance as a locus of LGBTQ community activism, results in feelings of frustration and alienation because for them, an HIV+ status and its attendant physical, emotional, and social ramifications still structure much of their everyday lives.

This disarticulation between contemporary hegemonic HIV/AIDS narratives that, for the most part, circulate unproblematically through Toronto HASOs and LGBTQ media, and memories of suffering and activism in the early decades of the AIDS epidemic, ongoing physical challenges stemming from HIV-related illnesses and earlier generations of toxic medications, and ongoing experiences of discrimination and rejection based on an HIV+ status, produces what I have called queer viral time, which for this group is a time out of joint, a time "out" of hetero- and homonormative timeframes, that is, distinct and disconnected from most present-day narratives of HIV/AIDS. However, I have also argued that there is no singular or collective queer viral time, and the comments from some members of this group about the increasing diversity of PLHIV in Toronto and the "problem" of HASOS paying more attention to "women, people on drugs and immigrants" reflect a particular assemblage of queer viral time premised on a homogenous gender, sexual, age, and racial orientations which reflect particular arrangements of privilege and marginalization.

This group's shared sense of queer viral time renders a temporal disjuncture between what "should be" and what "is," disrupting hegemonic narratives of HIV governance, subjectification, and discipline. It forms a critique of the ways in which aging is framed in much of the HIV/AIDS research, policy, and treatment practice as a biomedical problem of comorbidities and mental health issues that can be solved through "successful aging" strategies emphasizing individualized actions focusing on resilience, self-care, and generativities. These men's comments acknowledge (albeit indirectly) how this neoliberal, biopolitical framing of aging and living with HIV contributes to the fracturing and dismantling of queer community networks that have long served as a resource for care (Fitzgerald et al. 2019). Their anachronic sensibilities thus disrupt the smooth surface of "end of crisis" and "HIV as chronic illness" narratives and demonstrate the need for further examination of the biopolitics of time embedded in categories of health and illness in order to better understand the complex and changing realities for those living in queer viral time.

NOTES

1. This chapter was previously published in Murray, David AB. "Opting Out: Aging Gays, HIV/AIDS and the Bio-Politics of Queer Viral Time." *Journal of Homosexuality* (2021): 1–18.

2. https://www.unaids.org/en/topic/treatment accessed October 16, 2019

3. PrEP stands for preexposure prophylaxis and is an HIV prevention method in which people who don't have HIV take HIV medicine daily to reduce their risk of getting HIV if they are exposed to the virus. See below for further explanation of this group's perspectives on PrEP.

4. At my first group meeting, I informed members that I was conducting research on the topic of long-term PLHIV experiences of Toronto HASOs and sought permission to take notes on group meetings. Members provided their permission for note-taking as long as principles of confidentiality and anonymity were respected. Therefore, all names and any identifying features of participants mentioned in this chapter have been changed.

5. Age and racial identification are based on my observations, so perceptive bias may be an issue. HIV status and sexual orientation were self-declared by group members in various discussions and comments.

6. This group's perception of Toronto HASOs as increasingly bureaucratic and professionalized institutions echoes the findings of Cain et al.'s research focusing on challenges to the involvement of PLHIV in community-based HIV/AIDS organizations in Ontario, Canada (2014).

7. See, for example, the Canadian AIDS Treatment Information Exchange: https://www.catie.ca/en/fact-sheets/prevention/pre-exposure-prophylaxis-prep (accessed December 4, 2019).

8. Azidothymidine or AZT was one of the first medications found to be somewhat effective in controlling HIV and was approved by the Federal Drug Administration for distribution in 1987. However, AZT had severe side effects and was considered by some HIV activists to be more toxic than the virus itself. After the advent of more effective ART medications in the mid-1990s, reliance on AZT dropped substantially. https://time.com/4705809/first-aids-drug-azt/ (accessed December 4, 2019).

9. It should be noted that current research on PrEP indicates there are few long-term side effects, and that PrEP is therefore much less toxic than earlier generations of HIV medications like AZT. https://www.aidsmap.com/about-hiv/what-are-side-effects-truvada-used-prep (accessed November 11, 2020).

10. See note 9.

11. See Marshall et al. (2019) for a discussion of "queer generations" that similarly challenges the temporal assumptions of normative generational frameworks.

REFERENCES

AIDS Committee of Toronto (ACT). 2018. http://www.actoronto.org/health-information/people-living-with-hiv, accessed January 4, 2018.

Benton, Adia, Thurka Sangaramoorthy and Ippolytos Kalofonos. 2017. "Temporality and Positive Living in the Age of HIV/AIDS: A Multisited Ethnography." *Current Anthropology* 58, no.4: 454–476.

Boseley, Sarah and Hannah Devline. 2019. "End to AIDS in sight as huge study finds drugs stop HIV transmission." *The Guardian*, May 2. https://www.theguardian.com/society/2019/may/02/end-to-aids-in-sight-as-huge-study- finds-drugs-stop-hiv-transmission_

Cain, Roy, Evan Collins, Tarik Bereket, Clemon George, Randy Jackson, Alan Lie, Tracey Prentice and Robb Travers. 2014. "Challenges to the involvement of people living with HIV in community-based HIV/AIDS organizations in Ontario, Canada." *AIDS Care* 26, no. 2: 263–266, http://dx.doi.org/10.1080/09540121.2013.803015

CATIE (Canadian AIDS Treatment Information Exchange) 2010. *HIV and Aging*. Toronto: CATIE.

CATIE (Canadian AIDS Treatment Information Exchange) 2016. "Going Beyond Current Ideas about the Cascade of HIV Care." CATIE News, December 21, 2016. http://www.catie.ca/en/catienews/2016-12-21/going-beyond-current-ideas-about-cascade- hiv-care. Accessed December 23, 2016.

Colvin, Christopher J. 2011. "HIV/AIDS, chronic diseases and globalization." *Global Health* 7, no. 31. https://globalizationandhealth.biomedcentral.com/articles/10.1186/1744-8603-7-31

City of Toronto, Medical Officer of Health. 2015. *HIV in Toronto: Closing the Diagnosis Gap*. City of Toronto. No. 2.3.

Edelman, Lee. 2004. *No Future: Queer Theory and the Death Drive*. Durham. Duke University Press.

Farmer, Paul. 1999/2001. *Infections and Inequalities: The Modern Plagues*. Berkeley, CA: University of California Press.

Farmer, Paul. 2003. *Pathologies of Power: Health, Human Rights and the New War on the Poor*. Berkeley, CA: University of California Press.

Fitzgerald, Lisa, Cris Howard, Lisa Herron, Kate Hannan, Andrea Whittaker, and Alison Mutch. 2019. "'Is It HIV or Just Old Age?' How Australia's First Generation of PLHIV Are Experiencing Ageing." *HIV Australia*, June 6.

Government of Canada. 2016. *Global AIDS Response Progress Report: Canada 2016*. http://www.unaids.org/sites/default/files/country/documents/CAN_narrative_report_2016 .pdf. Accessed December 24, 2016.

Halbertam, J. Jack. 2005. *In a Queer Time and Place: Transgender Bodies, Subcultural Lives*. New York: New York University Press.

Halkitis, Peter. 2013. *The AIDS Generation: Stories of Survival and Resilience*. Oxford: Oxford University Press.

Hoad, Neville. 2007. *African Intimacies: Race, Homosexuality, and Globalization*. Minneapolis: University of Minnesota Press.

Jolivétte, Andrew. 2016. *Indian Blood: HIV and Colonial Trauma in San Francisco's Two-Spirit Community*. Seattle: University of Washington Press.

Leahy, Bob. 2017. "Ottawa's Envision Forum from Bruce House highlighted major issues facing aging HIVers." *Positive Lite*, March 29. http://www.positivelite.com/index.php/item/ottawa-s-envisionforum-from-bruce-house- highlighted-major-issues-facing-aging-hivers?category_id=100 (accessed January 13, 2018)

Lemke, Thomas. 2010. "From state biology to the government of life: Historical dimensions and contemporary perspectives of 'biopolitics.'" *Journal of Classical Sociology* 10, no. 4: 421–438.

Manderson, Lenore, and Caroline Smith-Morris, C. 2010. *Chronic conditions, fluid states: Chronicity and the Anthropology of Illness*. New Brunswick, NJ: Rutgers University Press.

Marshall, Daniel, Aggleton, P., Cover, C., Rasmussen, M. L., and Hegarty, B. 2019. "Queer generations: Theorizing a concept." *International Journal of Cultural Studies,* 22, no. 4, 558–576.

Mattes, Dominik. 2014. "Caught in transition: The struggle to live a 'normal' life with HIV in Tanzania." *Medical Anthropology* 33, 270–287.

McCaskell, Tim. 2006. "Power to the People: A look back at the issues, struggles and victories that defined the early age of AIDS activism in Canada." *The Positive Side*. Spring/Summer. https://www.catie.ca/en/positiveside/springsummer-2006/power-people

McDonald, Karalyn, Julian Elliott, and Lise Saugeres. 2013. "Ageing with HIV in Victoria: Findings from a Qualitative Study." *HIV Australia* 11, no. 2, 13–16.

McKinley, Jesse. 2019. "New York Says End of AIDS Epidemic Is Near." *The New York Times*, October 2. Accessed October 15, 2019. https://www.nytimes.com/2019/10/02/nyregion/aids-hiv-epidemic-ny.html

Moyer, Eileen. 2015. "The anthropology of life after AIDS: Epistemological continuities in the age of antiretroviral treatment." *Annual Review of Anthropology* 44:259–75.

Ontario HIV Epidemiology and Surveillance Initiative (OHESI). 2019. *New HIV diagnoses in Ontario, 2017.* Toronto, Ontario. http://www.ohesi.ca/reports-data/ Accessed December 6, 2019.

Ontario HIV Treatment Network. 2012. *Evidence Informing the Intersection of HIV, Aging and Health - A scoping review.* https://www.google.com/url?sa=t&rct=j&q=&esrc=s&source=web&cd=1&ved=2ahUKEwjA7ZKsh5rmAhUPpFkKHRRLCQcQFjAAegQIBBAC&url=http%3A%2F%2Fwww.ohtn.on.ca%2FDocuments%2FResearch%2FOHTN-Positive-Aging-Final-Report-2012-12.pdf&usg=AOvVaw3k9kTMCBAWOVAcs4xGa91j Accessed December 4, 2019.

Patton, Cindy. 2002. *Globalizing AIDS*. Minneapolis: University of Minnesota Press.

Sangaramoorthy, Thurka. 2014. *Treating AIDS: Politics of Difference, Paradox of Prevention* New Brunswick, NJ: Rutgers University Press.

Sangaramoorthy, Thurka. 2018. "Chronicity, Crisis and the 'End of AIDS.'" *Global Public Health* 13, no. 1: 1–15.

Stockdill, Brett. 2003. *Activism against AIDS: At the Intersection of Sexuality, Race, Gender, and Class*. Boulder: Lynne Rienner Publishers.

UNAIDS. 2013. *HIV and Aging*. A special supplement to the UNAIDS report on the global AIDS epidemic 2013. Geneva: unaids.org

UNAIDS. 2016. UNAIDS Programme Coordinating Board. "HIV and ageing." UNAIDS/PCB (39)/16.25 Issue date: 14 November 2016.

Chapter 8

From "At-Risk" to Interdependent

The Erotic Life Worlds of HIV+ Jamaican Women

Jallicia Jolly

"*Mi*[1] *nuh know bout you but mi nuh sick!*" ["I don't know about you, but I'm not sick!"][2] exclaims Donna—a 24-year-old HIV+ community organizer and working-class mother of one during a conversation about relationships, sex, and illness with a group of other young HIV+ women.[3] She is a dark-skinned, single mother from Spanish Town, her hometown, the capital city of the neighboring parish St. Catherine, and the second largest town in Jamaica. Her eyebrows raised and finger wagged as she reenacted an internal dialogue she had during a recent intimate encounter with a male partner. She exclaimed: "*If mi nuh feel like mi wan tell yuh [mi HIV status], weh yuh tink mi do? Mi mek sure seh mi wear fucking condoms!*" ["If I don't feel like I want to tell you [my HIV status], what do you think I do? I make sure I use fucking condoms!"]. Donna continued by sharing the ways she reconciled her desires for intimate connection and sexual fulfillment while living with a socially stigmatizing, physically deteriorating, and emotionally debilitating marker that is potentially lethal (Watkins-Hayes 2008). Participating in the youth-friendly, women-centered networks of EVE for Life (EFL)—Jamaica's first HIV psychosocial support and advocacy organization for HIV+ young mothers as well as girls and women who experience sexual violence—served to rejuvenate Donna's desire to live despite her stigmatized embodiment. The affective communion that Donna shared with other women enabled her to contest the exclusionary boundaries of social belonging and political organizing and leadership around HIV.

Donna's obligations as an organizer and mentor of other young HIV+ women form a broader trajectory of her self-discovery. Diagnosed with HIV during the pregnancy of her first child in 2011, Donna describes then entering a dark period where she felt like "*mi dead now!*" [I am dead now!]. Within four years of joining EFL, Donna has established herself as a professional mentor to several women in her Spanish Town community who have recently been diagnosed with HIV or who lack the proper knowledge to protect themselves. In many ways, she has reconstructed her life, focusing on her work in HIV and youth empowerment in urban communities, raising her four-year-old daughter, and working as a peer mentor as she takes free leadership and business classes at a local training institution supported by an international development agency. Often viewed in her neighborhood as a sex educator, Donna is called upon community members and friends to provide condoms and advice about relationships and sex.

In various ways, Donna's participation in EFL's psychosocial support groups and her community health work with other HIV+ women have fostered interdependent communities of care and belonging. Importantly, they counter the ongoing neglect of culturally appropriate approaches to HIV among marginalized Black women. This is but one example of the important role of women-centered networks in the intimate life and health activism of young Black women, and the ways in which they allow women to articulate ideas about intimacy, community building, and bodily autonomy that are relevant to their daily needs. The women-led space of EFL and its ascendance as an HIV women's organization with transnational and diasporic dimensions produces social intimacies that heighten racial and gender consciousness as they cultivate homosocial networks of care.[4] For HIV+ Black Caribbean women, questions of health and sickness as well as exclusion and marginalization implicate intimacy in uncomfortable matters of global inequities and illness. These questions complicate how women interpret their diagnosis and experience sex and sexuality. Importantly, they also deeply inform the process by which women become conscious of their social position as HIV+ people who are politically active by maintaining different institutional ties and performing overlapping roles as community organizers, public speakers, advocates, and peer educators known as "Mentor Moms" and "Mentee Moms."[5] To date, the political uses of women's intimacies in relation to HIV in public health discourses remain underexamined and largely ignored.

The collectivity displayed by EFL participants like Donna presents a striking contrast to the public HIV/AIDS care model that prioritizes individualism, self-help, and self-sufficiency in "end of crisis" narratives circulated by global health organizations such as USAIDS, UNAIDS, and GFTAM.[6] Traditional prevention and treatment strategies have long emphasized the path to the "End of AIDS" which describes the lofty goal of eliminating all clinical disease and death due to HIV infection.[7] This goal is driven by UN's Fast Track 90-90-90 targets for 2020, which aims to provide strong global targets and indicators by which to measure progress within national HIV/AIDS strategic plans. Yet, this individualistic public health approach has often neglected an understanding of the interlocking forms of social stratification integral to the experience of illness in Jamaica. Jamaica's increasing reliance on aid from the United States, Germany, and other countries within the European Union also stems from long-standing challenges of postcolonial Jamaica's experience with debt and structural adjustment policies that led to reductions in government health care expenditures, privatization of medical care, and underemployment. While these forces have provided funding and resources that established a public access program for antiretroviral (ARV) treatment of persons with AIDS and advanced HIV, they have also crystallized priority areas and populations, which continue to exclude Black women. The absence of meaningful support structures and global investments in women in the Global South in general, and Black women in particular, requires a need for greater focus on the unique ways women live and organize while grappling with overlapping forms of oppression and managing illness and HIV care.

Even as Black feminist scholarship and artistry have long engaged Black women's intimate lives, there is limited work on the disproportionate impact of HIV and AIDS on Black girls and women, especially those in non-US contexts.[8] The past few decades of the pandemic have seen a radical transformation in biomedical interventions and a relative increase in new funding schemes and initiatives of international organizations, agencies, and governments of more resourced countries in North America and Europe (Moyer 2015). Yet, in the Caribbean region and in Jamaica, the uneven distribution of resources for HIV prevention for women, a population often framed as a nonpriority, remains a glaring erasure in local and global initiatives. As current models emphasize approaches that advocate targeting the behaviors of specific groups known as "high-risk" or "key populations" such as "men who have sex with men (MSM)" and "sex workers," programs and research have yet to garner complete understandings of the intricate sexual and social dynamics that can make them effectively reduce HIV among nonnormative groups such as Black gay men, trans women, Black girls and women.[9] Furthermore, such particularistic agendas conflate sexual orientation with sexual practices, which ignores the spectrum of intimate exchanges among various individuals, thereby rendering many HIV interventions targeting young women ineffective. As a result, the sociocultural realities of HIV-positive women remain underexamined, and little is known about the life-worlds that give rise to the everyday knowledge and intimate connections women employ to develop and sustain community-driven actions that contest gender inequalities and stigmatization associated with the disease.

In this feminist ethnography of HIV+ women's intimate and political lives in Kingston, Jamaica, I delineate how women in activist organizations develop and cultivate HIV/AIDS care strategies through women-centered networks. I read these networks as intentional communities of interdependence and psychosocial care, rather than simply invisible "at-risk" groups or passive victims subjected to "a paralyzing plague." I contend that the homosocial intimacies that characterize these networks of care reflect an "intraventive" cultural practice and knowledge, a term that Marlon Bailey uses to describe the organic ways community members represent themselves individually and collectively (Bailey, 2013, 183, 203–204). I use the concept of the erotic to allude to women's grassroots politics and their self-making practices through mentorship networks, support groups, and dancehall spaces which, in the context of intersecting forces, managed to enable affective connections and pleasure that repurpose discourses of shame and disease into calls for interdependence and resistance. Women's experiences point to a tripartite conception of the erotic that embraces the interlinkage among political work, sensual desire, and sacred connections, which inform women's formation of interdependent social networks and their navigations of marginalization and inequality.[10] By foregrounding the erotic as an embodied resource that gives rise to new kinds of political projects centered on self- and community-care, I show how women navigate inequality and disrupt narratives of HIV/AIDS progress that obscure the power relations that undermine their well-being. The politics of the erotic and illness reveal how the embodied knowledges of HIV+ Black women challenge pathologizing public health and academic discourses, while also serving as conduits for enhancing and extending theories about bodies, sexuality, power, and intimacy. By offering a culturally specific exploration of the socioerotic lives of working-class HIV+ Jamaican women, this chapter concludes with a discussion about how centering our analysis on Caribbean and Black women expands the geographic and thematic scopes of studies of race, sexuality, and HIV/AIDS.

I use the erotic to describe how illness can cultivate a range of intimacies that become a form of Black feminist agency and community building through support groups, mentorship relationships, and grassroots community activities.[11] By leveraging the multidimensional dimensions of the erotic in Black Caribbean women's lives, I embrace Lamonda Horton-Stallings's use of culturally specific Afrocentric concepts such as "funk" and "stank" to describe the Black body in labor and to foreground pleasure and community that transcends forms of discipline and structures of biopower.[12] My use of the term describes how women's lives generate knowledge about the everyday uses of sexuality that enable them to use their bodies as tools for connection, pleasure, support, and mobilization. This form of epistemic practice is designed not only to resist the ignorance about HIV and other STDs by providing accessible medical knowledge but also to encourage women to learn their own bodies and sexualities in order to protect their health while affirming their desires and aspirations. As active sites of knowledge production and dissemination, HIV+ Jamaican women's bodies and relationships with each other reveal their embodied knowledge as an instructive social and political resource that enables a radical representation of women on their own terms.

I locate my understanding of the critical links between the erotic and illness in women's lives within recent Caribbean and Black feminist scholarship on sexuality, pleasure, and abjection. As this recent work evolved expansive visions of Black women's sexual politics and Black sexual subjectivity, sites of abjection—the repulsive and undisciplined—became grounds to model new subject positions, unsettle cultural ideals, and transform rigid norms of gender and sexuality.[13] For example, Mimi Sheller (2012) elaborates on a "citizenship from below" which contextualizes how subaltern Caribbean sexual subjects appear, are silenced, and contest and/or reproduce hegemonic perspectives. Gloria Wekker's notion of "mati work" provides fertile ground to engage the specificities of working-class Afro-Caribbean women's bodies and sexual practices beyond the normative sensibilities of Euro-American heterosexuality (2006). Jennifer Nash's concept of "ecstasy" (2014) and Mireille Miller-Young's notion of "brown sugar" (2013) provide incisive examinations of the performative dimensions of Black women's sexual labor in ways that develop radical notions of bodies and sexual intimacy. Similarly, Juana Maria Rodriguez (2014), Lamonda Horton-Stallings (2015), Rosamond King (2014), and Jacqui Alexander's (1994) discussions about the radical implications of women's outlaw sexuality help intervene in paternalist social and political contexts. I use this body of work to uncover tensions between the erotic, subjectivity, and colonial racial and sexual inequalities. Building on this opening, I further explore how differently located women in various cultural contexts negotiate political claims alongside their pursuits for erotic connections beyond the pathologizing impulses of state and institutional forces.

Rarely are Black women, especially those who are poor, working class, and HIV+, considered leaders of social and political movements, much less political theorists in official discourses. Yet, Caribbean theorists and activists have long engaged the gendered and sexual possibilities of both women's cultural and political movements. While HIV+ Black women have been at the very heart of struggles in the hemisphere for quality HIV care and against intersectional forms of structural vulnerabilities that heighten women's emotional, psychic, and sexual trauma, they remain excluded in political discourses and academic scholarship on HIV activist history and Black political movements. Looking to the political action and intimate practices in the daily lives of Black Caribbean women will offer sociocultural models for how to live with, organize around, and prevent HIV/AIDS. Importantly, this focus deepens the cultural knowledge of Black women's contributions to the transnational political dimensions of the pandemic, which can reveal ways to leverage the labor and networks of activists and grassroots organizations to reduce the racial and gendered disparities of HIV/AIDS.

This work is animated and enabled by my own subject position as a young black woman and a Jamaican American scholar. My complexly constituted social and political positionality facilitated both my entry into the scenes illustrated throughout this chapter and my ongoing relationships and interactions with interlocutors. This entrance embraces Rosamond King and Angelique Nixon's use of the concept of "embodied theories" (2013) as a feminist methodology that acknowledges the materiality and affect of the body as well as the spatial and intellectual location of the scholar while being respectful and responsive to the communities we study. It is this complex "diasporic outsider-within subjectivity" that has guided my navigation of compounded erasures as I work to address the inattention to Black women in general, and Caribbean women in particular in studies of Black politics, gender, and HIV/AIDS; to decenter the United States in studies of racialized sexuality, power, and inequality in the Americas; and to illuminate the significance of HIV+ Black Caribbean women's lives to intellectual and political work that connects racial, gender, and sexual justice more concretely (Allen, 2012, 326; Harrison 1991, 2009). My own status as HIV– further informs this "outsider-within subjectivity" as it has shaped the privilege I have accessed and leveraged to navigate state institutions, organizations, and public spaces with HIV+ women. It is through these embodied differences that I intimately experience how Black women's bodies accentuate the continual struggle between the subject and the abject, the normal and the deviant.

EXPANDING THEORIES OF INTERSECTIONALITY AND HIV/AIDS

As women's experiences reveal, an ethnographic study of the intimate lives of HIV+ Black Caribbean women extends theories of sexuality, intimacy, and the body in three primary ways. First, it empirically studies how intersectionality unfolds in the lives of Black women living with and impacted by HIV and AIDS, which augments the mostly theoretical analyses of Black women's sexualities and agency. In addition to adding the lived realities of Black women to the ethnographic record, it brings into focus the political significance of the Caribbean in studies of Black politics, sexual cultures, and health. And finally, it demonstrates how illness and racialized sexuality matter to the body and quotidian life, shaping women's physical and psychic realities as well as their relations with and among other women. Collectively, these contributions spotlight a reservoir of cultural interventions too often revoked of legibility in mainstream scholarship and movements.

Recent scholarship on race, gender, and sexuality has used intersectionality as a framework to illustrate how illness and marginalization matter to Black sexual politics. Cathy Cohen's (1997) canonical study of how cultural elites and political figures used the stigma of HIV/AIDS to internalize and replicate racial, gendered, and class hierarchies within African American communities revealed the diverse responses to highly moralized AIDS discourses.[14] Additionally, political scientist Michelle Tracy Berger uses the concept of "intersectional stigma" to offer a model of how to empirically study how marginalization constrains Black and Latina women's access to resources and services, ultimately shaping their health trajectories and political participation (Berger, 2004, 24–25). Marlon Bailey's ethnographic exploration of the performance of racialized, gender, sex, and sexuality in the development of agentive responses to HIV uses the body as a site to develop expansive ways to study the culturally specific expressions of sexuality and desire. According to Lyndon Gill's discussion of queer Afro-Trinidadian men's community organizing, the intimacy of activism is a galvanizing political, social, and sensual force in an array of relationships among male participants in a local organization. The radical "uses of desire" and sensuality are evident as HIV+ and HIV– queer Afro-Trinidadians explore their sexual desires and social intimacies through "touch" as opposed to the chaos-inducing rhetoric of contagion (Gill 2018, 176). Similarly, Darius Bost's exploration of the Black gay cultural renaissance through Black gay men's literary and cultural work reveals a legacy of their deliberate sociality and community building that contests their portrayal as illegible victims in the face of antiblackness and antiqueerness. It is precisely this insistence on holistic living and community that foregrounds my documentation of Black women's movement building through their embodied connections and political claims. It is this investment in new vocabularies of intimacy and sexuality that bolsters Donna's opening statement: "*Mi nuh sick!*" ["I'm not sick!"]. Like other women, she is invested in a sensual activism that moves beyond the exclusive emphasis on contagion and disclosure in HIV interventions, which allows women to pursue interdependent relationships and desires that emerge in their networks.

This expansive engagement with intersectionality activates my discussion of both Black women's embodied experiences and their relation to institutional, legal, and social forces that enable their invisibility and vulnerability (Nash 2019). Collectively, these works collapse the divisions between Black politics and Black sexuality, demonstrating how HIV necessitates more complete analyses of Afro-diasporic communities and the ways in which these communities have responded to seemingly disparate spheres of the sexual and the political.[15] Amid the lack of qualitative studies of HIV that center ethnographic approaches, a culturally rooted and empirically driven account of HIV+ Black women's subaltern ways of knowing can help unpack the nuanced intersections of racialized gender, sexual, and class differences in the experience of illness and marginalization.[16] As the claims of Donna and other women demonstrate, these counter modes of intimacy and self-presentation offer possibilities for marginalized women to carve out space for self-making beyond the delimited sites of public health and HIV advocacy that emphasize respectability and individual self-sufficiency. Furthermore, an intersectional ethnographic methodology complicates dominant HIV narratives by documenting how the daily textures of women's lives and embodied realities upend their unidimensional portrayals as static, passive, and vulnerable objects in 'end of AIDS' discourses. This contextual and empirically driven account foregrounds how interlocking components of race, gender, class, and sexuality are neglected in crises narrative that ignore how these dynamics shape how women mediate notions of difference, self, community, and health while facing economic and social challenges.

WOMEN AND HIV/AIDS IN THE CARIBBEAN

Donna's opening statement and life story highlight aspects of the lived experiences of a population that is increasingly impacted by HIV—young Black women between the ages of 15 and 26 (Whiteside 2008, 8). Globally, AIDS-related illnesses remain the leading cause of death for women of reproductive age, and those ages 15–24 years account for a disproportionate number of new infections (Whiteside 2008, 21). Even though the Caribbean has both the highest incidence rates of reported AIDS cases and HIV prevalence rates in the Americas, second only to Africa, little is known about the region's significance in curtailing the scourge of HIV/AIDS in Black communities globally. Although Jamaica was touted as an emerging Caribbean HIV success story in the early 2000s, in recent years, it has faced high prevalence rates among "MSM," transgender men and women, and "low-risk heterosexual" women.[17] Girls between the ages of 15 and 19 are three times more likely to be infected than boys their age, while women aged 20–24 are one and a half times more likely to be infected than men in the same age group.[18] These historic trends align with existing data on HIV prevalence in Jamaica that shows that girls and women living with HIV increased dramatically from 30% of reported cases between 1980 and 1989 to 46% between 2009 and 2012.[19] These trends also highlight the growing disconnect between technological and medical advances and disease burden among Afro-diasporic women, which invites further exploration of the intimate racial and sexual dynamics that mediate HIV's impact on women's everyday lives.

That young Black women are disproportionately represented in the global rates of HIV and AIDS is not a phenomenon unique to Jamaica. Working-class women throughout the African diaspora maintain a structurally disadvantaged position in comparison with people within non-Western and Western contexts in ways that play out in the domains of sexuality and health. Recent scholarship on gender inequality and HIV/AIDS has demonstrated how structural inequalities and women's economic dependence on men reconfigure the social landscape of HIV risk in ways that disproportionately impact women (Parikh 2007; White and Carr 2005; Farmer 2004). Collectively this work has aimed to understand HIV/AIDS organizing as "part of a broader process of social transformation, aimed not merely at the reduction of risk but at the redress of the social and economic inequality and injustice that has almost universally been found linked to increased vulnerability" to HIV and AIDS (Parker 2001). The marginal positions of women in the underclass and in the lower strata of the working class within both the economy and the political apparatus of the state reflect the gendered and racialized inequality of Jamaica's political economy (Wekker 2006). As Gina Ulysse notes, the enduring legacy of colonial racialization in contemporary Jamaican society creates deeply rooted racial and gender hierarchies that are color-coded and inflected upon the bodies of Black working-class women.[20] Within this context of class and color stratification, HIV, as both a medical condition and a sociocultural reality, plays a critical role in how women engage their embodiment, political agency, gender inequality, and general well-being in ways that demand greater understanding of how women's intimate lives evolve care practices and political strategies necessary for survival.

Two omissions impact the current dearth of research on Black women and HIV: the lack of culturally rooted explorations of Black sexual politics and Black women's sexualities in Black studies as well as the lack of interdisciplinary frameworks of race, gender, and sexuality in public health interventions and HIV prevention research. Black cultural studies scholars have continually noted how the lack of informed research and interventions on HIV/AIDS in Black communities contributes to the disproportionate rates of the pandemic among Black people in the United States. For example, Cathy Cohen's discussion of how disenfranchised groups respond to restrictive cultural mores revealed the failure of both Black elites and Black studies to address how HIV/AIDS and crosscutting issues—issues of identity that extend beyond race and that disproportionately affect certain segments of marginal groups—complicate societal privilege and oppression within racial and gender hierarchies (Cohen 1999, 9, 13–15). Patricia Hill Collins observed that these issues raised by the HIV epidemic suggest the need to move beyond the restrictive emphasis on "individual risk" and toward progressive understandings of Black sexual politics that engender new conceptualizations of body politics, relationships, and community (Collins 2004, 296). Yet, few efforts leverage Black studies as a site of cultural inquiry to address the Black AIDS pandemic because of the ongoing distance between academic researchers and community and divisions between theoretical and practical knowledge (Cohen 1999, 27; Bailey 2009, 255).

It is precisely because of the deep familiarity of Afro-diasporic people with stigmatized embodiment and Black studies with challenging hierarchies of knowledge that we must heed these clarion calls to explore the gendered, racial, and sexual dimensions of HIV. Additionally, because Afro-Caribbeans, specifically Haitians, were the only ethnic groups viewed inherently susceptible to the disease, it is imperative to engage the Black Caribbean in these discussions about the cultural practices used to trouble dominant AIDS discourses and practices.[21]

The Caribbean and Latin American studies literature on adolescents and HIV has represented youth sexuality in the region as problematic, socially pathological, and politically deficient. Kamala Kempadoo, Oneka LaBennett, and numerous others have critiqued this social science approach to the intimate lives of young Black women who are often described as "at-risk" for social, psychological, and physical problems such as teenage pregnancy, drug use, and participation in violent crime (Kempadoo 2009; LaBennett 2011). This assumed degeneracy frames women as "carriers of disease," which eludes the structural, global, and quotidian dynamics that shape their perceptions of and responses to inequality and HIV/AIDS. In Jamaica, public health discourses and research frame young women through conversations about the early sexual initiation of girls, poor women as "vectors of disease" responsible for the spread of HIV to men and their children, and transactional sexual relationships as public health problems and reproductive health concerns. The hypervisibility of Black Jamaican women's bodies and sexualities works in tandem with their invisibility as subjects worthy of political recognition, opportunities for social mobility, health resources, and related investments in well-being. Even though Jamaica has both a generalized HIV epidemic in the population and a concentrated epidemic among specific populations such as queer men, sex workers, and young women, women's label as "nonkey populations" denies them access to critical funding sources for prevention work, research, and HIV-related services.[22]

Pathological descriptions of the intimate lives of girls and women emphasize Caribbean feminist Kamala Kempadoo's observation that the reductionist biases in HIV and AIDS have undermined more complete understandings of the social and political lives of Caribbean youth (Kempadoo 2009, 11). I heed Kempadoo's clarion call to interrogate the "uncritical problematization" of Caribbean youth's "sexual praxis," which she describes as "the ways in which sexuality is made visible through behaviors, activities and interactions between people, in relations, and in the ways in which desires are actualized."[23] This expansive focus challenges the surveillance and regulation of marginalized Black youth as it intervenes in the elisions in sexual health research and HIV prevention studies by articulating Caribbean youth's agency and desires beyond traditional narratives of innocent children or deviant young adults.[24]

As Jamaica becomes part of a global network of low- and middle-income countries that comprise the growing share of the global HIV/AIDS burden, more sophisticated analyses are needed to capture how the pandemic shapes ontological ways of being in the world and the range of bodily experiences in culturally inflected ways. The country's weakened health systems infrastructure has made the provision of prevention services and resources for treatment and care challenging. Growing socioeconomic inequalities further strengthen the country's dependency on international aid organizations to implement public health and social welfare programs. For example, the Global Fund to Fight AIDS, Tuberculosis and Malaria (GFATM) has facilitated the country's initial expansion of HIV prevention efforts, which enabled the implementation of HIV treatment and prevention and the development of educational access programs for ARV treatment for people living with HIV and AIDS in 2004. The President's Emergency Plan for AIDS Relief (PEPFAR) has provided resources to support large-scale prevention, treatment, and care against AIDS, malaria, and tuberculosis. The recent investments of GFATM of $14.9 million for 2016–2018 and PEPFAR of $5 million for 2015–2016 have strengthened the roles of these international agencies as critical players in the country's civic and social processes.[25] Beyond its typical framing as a site of global networks of tourism and travel, Jamaica, and the Caribbean more generally, are cultural spheres that are not new to either imposed cultural and economic agendas or transnational forces and circuits of ideas about Blackness. Ultimately, the growing influence of global health organizations often gives donors and agencies increasing power to shape the agendas of local organizations, women's lives, and their access to care and political opportunities.[26]

The transformative work of Caribbean feminist organizations has emerged in this space. Founded in Kingston in 2008 by two Jamaican women, Patricia Watson and Joy Crawford, EFL emerged in this complex terrain of health and inequality during the years when women shouldered the highest numbers of AIDS-related death.[27] The exclusion of women in HIV care and aid was the impetus for the local actors and leaders of EFL to implement interventions for young women living with HIV and AIDS. As the product of growing efforts to expand the gendered dimensions of the national HIV/AIDS response during the 1990s, EFL provides a continuum of psychosocial care and support services that includes gender-specific services of the Mentor Mom Initiative (MMI). This initiative uses mentorship between women who are newly diagnosed and those who have been living with HIV for a longer time to meet the developmental and health needs of women and girls. In particular, the program remains a national model for holistic approaches to HIV and a key part of EFL's cross-regional, cross-sectoral, and intergenerational organizing work. Buttressed by their connection to the local public health system and community clinics, EFL has been successful at reaching working-class, underemployed, and unemployed urban Black Jamaican women. They are not only inadequately attended to by the vast majority of the nation's health care and HIV/AIDS-related initiatives but are also overrepresented in populations needing the sexual and reproductive health services of the underresourced public health system. EFL's grassroots origin is sustained through its community work with the MMI, which continues to be a collective space for mentorship, intergenerational knowledge sharing, training, and resource sharing among its participants.

A POLITICS OF INTERDEPENDENCE: HOLISTIC CARE BEYOND MERE SURVIVAL

As a Mentor Mom of the Kingston chapter of EFL at the time of the interview, Donna suggested that the relationships developed among women expanded the nature of HIV prevention work that overemphasized disease progression and medical terms. She states further: "Wi did want fi help people live, jus coz being HIV+ yuh nuh dead. Yuh see, coz we formulate around young ooman, it's like it give wi di drive. It start fi give me drive when mi see di things dem do. Dem did do sex ed way, way differently, and not only dat, but wid younga people. We affi show dem dat dis cyan happen, yuh know, but yuh still cyan smile . . . and people are here fi help yuh get thru it." ["We [wanted] to help people live, just because being HIV+ you are not dead. You see, [because] we formulate around young women, it's like it gives us the drive. . . . It started to give me drive when I saw the things they were doing. . . . They were doing sex ed way, way differently, and not only that, but with younger people. We have to show them that this can happen, you know, but you still can smile . . . and people are here to help you get through it."]

The MMI of the EFL organization challenges current hegemonic HIV/AIDS discourses because it is steeped in a rich cultural context of community care that embraces the value of interdependence and psychosocial care in the face of coercion, stigma, and social exclusion.[28] In practice, these values and commitments revolve around a circular model of care and support that is based on the work of staff and participants who are "Mentor moms"—educators of HIV and sexual reproductive health—and "Mentee moms"—newly diagnosed women and students in training. The Mentor Mom program remains paramount in the body of EFL's work and serves as a mechanism for EFL to assess and address the particular needs of teenage mothers and young adult women, its capacity to meet those needs, and the nature of its relationship with communities most in need amid declining funding streams for HIV care. Its presence as a social site and political entity has bound women in intergenerational relationships where they could convene and connect in similarly oriented communities. This relational model for understanding women's experience with illness has become a central organizing mechanism that generates interpersonal relations, desires, and emotional states which have formed the basis of collective relationships.

As Donna described how her entrance into the community of women at the EFL organization fostered her drive to actively participate in a leadership role, she reveals how her health status and intimate connections to other women catalyzed her self-definition while cultivating her organizational ties. This fellowship with other HIV+ women similarly committed to community health work around HIV awareness and reproductive health education also extended beyond the space of EFL. Mentor Moms also provided support for HIV prevention among HIV– women by leading educational workshops at local prenatal clinics. In a vivid retelling of the affirmative reception of the workshop by clinic attendees, Donna notes: "How we did do [condom demonstration], people enjoyed it, even di oral [demonstration] and odda tings . . . [Ooman] don't discuss oral sex so when wi start dweet and show we did tr fi bring it out, and they were like, 'Fi real! Luk how she dweet, look how dat girl put on condoms!' Some people didn't even know seh there were female condoms." ["How we did [condom demonstration], people enjoyed it, even the oral [demonstration] and other things. . . . [Women] don't discuss oral sex so when we started to do it and show we tried to bring it out, and they were like, 'For real! Look how she do it, look how that girl put on condoms!' Some people didn't even know there were female condoms."]

Beyond the sexual health workshops, a politicized form of community building emerges in the interdependent communities of HIV+ Jamaican women that incorporate care for self, care for other women, and care for community. The role of interdependence in these articulations and expressions of care incorporates both professional obligations and informal care work. Donna remarked that her and her Mentee Mom, Tora, a 21-year-old mother of two, share a bond beyond the official provision of services outlined in her formal contract of Mentor Moms that involved both practical and intangible support for engagement in more holistic health-enhancing behaviors and practices. In my conversations with Donna and Tora, Tora often referenced how her relationship with Donna motivated her to survive: "When mi just know [EFL] . . . all through di day, Donna call mi fi ask me how mi ah do, when is mi clinic date. Dat is Donna . . . Donna find di time." ["When I just know [EFL] . . . all through the day, Donna called me [to] ask me how I am doing, when is my clinic date. That is Donna. Donna finds the time."]

The daughter of a single mother, Tora grew up in a low-income neighborhood in Spanish Town. As we spoke, her slim figure rested alongside the concrete barrier near the waterfront in Downtown Kingston. The sky was clear light blue painted with bright yellow rays. Coconut palm trees lined up along the busy downtown streets as we looked deep into the blue horizon. Her thick Black lashes rested along her deep-set brown eyes as she gazed at the letters "N-E-I-L" tattooed on her left index finger. With deep curiosity, I rested my eyes on the ink pasted on her flesh. Noticing my gaze, Tora remarked: "Mi shoulda leave him! Mi want scratch dis off!" ["I should leave him! I want to scratch this off!"]. I later learned that 'Neil' was short for Daniel, who was Tora's *babyfadda*, the father of her daughter and her on-and-off partner of four years. Tora's adolescence, what she described as "carefree," was shaped by her experiences of rape and forced transactional sex, as well as a tense and distant relationship with her mother. Diagnosed with HIV during the pregnancy of her first child in 2013, Tora described then entering a dark period: "After di docta tell mi mi have a new disease otha dan gonorrhea and was positive, mi did want fi run inna i road and mek one of di bus lick mi." [After the doctor told me I had a new disease other than gonorrhea and was positive, I wanted to run in the road and make one of the bus hit me.] She immediately disclosed to Neil and her mother, who encouraged her to "jus continue fi tek yuh pills dem" ["just continue to take your pills"]. Since then, she has become a Mentee Mom at EFL. During the time we first met in 2015, she worked a few days each week as a street cleaner—a job of many poor, darker-skinned Jamaicans. Tora is reframing her diagnosis while reconstructing a life in community with other women at EFL as she redevelops her relationship with Neil.

Tora describes care that involves not only encouraging adherence to medical and clinical appointments to reduce the threat of HIV progressing to AIDS and potentially death, but it also involves bodily, psychic, and emotional care that often addressed overlapping obstacles of unstable housing, underemployment, food insecurity, sexual violence, and stigma. These bonds often extended beyond the spaces of EFL and were connected to daily care activities such as caring for each other's children, sending reminders to take

ARV medication and to attend medical appointments, accompanying women to clinic visits, sensitizing family members and partners to HIV/AIDS, and even purchasing groceries and clothes. Clearly, care for the community binds women's care for self and care for each other as they saw their individual well-being and collective interests as closely linked to their community's access to psychosocial support, medical knowledge, and quality health services relevant to their quotidian needs.

EFL actors' antisexist work and struggles against gender oppression in approaches to the pandemic are reflective of the legacies of Caribbean and Black feminist organizations. The mobilization of activists rooted in explicit and implicit feminist consciousness accompanied by concrete action around basic needs and strategic interests forms part of a broader legacy of Black women's responses to marginalization throughout the diaspora (Springer 2005; Nixon and King 2013). The autonomous collective women created together cemented their commitments to broader communities where they lived and organized. This motivating factor undergirded their commitments to serve as educators and the longevity of the care labor they provided, especially during times when they worked without compensation.[29] The intimacy created by EFL actors in their care for the self, care for other women, and care for community evolved a politicized form of self-making and community building that provides the appropriate circumstances for the development of a radical politics of care from the ground up.

EMBODIED KNOWLEDGE: THE POLITICAL USES OF ILLNESSES

Star, an HIV+ 24-year-old woman at the time, approached a panel of international donors in the early morning on November 18, 2015, the 25th National HIV/STI Program's (NHP) Annual Review and Planning Retreat, which occurred in Montego Bay, Jamaica.[30] Following a presentation on the state of adolescence and HIV from Jamaica's Ministry of Health, Star boldly approached the mic and explained: "This [HIV] issue concerns me as a youth, one that has been raped, and is HIV+, and as a teen mother. . . . I think that getting the adolescents involved in policy making and being engaged with the issues because if it is not for us, you won't know the problems, you won't know how to solve them, how to go around it."

A wave of "mhmms" reverberated throughout the room as Star walked to her seat. Articulating her frustration with the often top-down nature of policy-making that is controlled by donors and the Government of Jamaica, her intervention highlights how she mobilizes her intersectional identity as an HIV+ woman, a youth, a mother, and a survivor of sexual violence in HIV organizing. Star is a Mentor Mother at the Montego Bay location of EFL who emerged as a prominent voice in the local HIV/AIDS community in the last five years. I met her one day during my visit to the Kingston location of EFL. She sat on the couch resting firmly on the peach-colored veranda. The smooth strands of her brown hair were slicked back in a low bun, stressing her glaring eyes and caramel brown skin. She was attentive and open as she introduced herself and her seven-year-old daughter, Shay. Shay's buoyant personality sharply contrasted her mother's calm demeanor. During our conversation she explained: "I started when I just had her. I was infected with HIV after being abused at age nine. My stepfather raped me. My mother didn't believe me. She said I was lying. My community blamed me for it and for shaming my stepfather. He died before my mother. He had it [HIV] too. I am not sure if she had it. I still don't know what killed her." My eyes widened as she recounted her story in one breath as Shay played in the distance. She continued: "Yeh, mi talk about dis all di time on TV and at conferences round di country. . . . She know about everything. Mi try nuh hide nuttin from har." ["Yeah, I talk about this all the time on TV and at conferences around the country. She knows about everything. I try not to hide anything from her."] Star smiled graciously.

Star's testimony at the NHP conference made it publicly clear that she, like many of the other women in EFL, has a keen awareness of the exclusions of HIV+ young women in the national response to HIV/AIDS. As a mother living with HIV and invested in full selfhood, Star embodies the sexual anxieties inscribed in the public health discourse of HIV as a moral panic and threat to the national health. Yet, as an HIV advocate and community organizer of EFL, Star's transformation journey represents the political possibilities that stem from her use of community health activism to intervene in public conversations that frame HIV+ women in general, and young mothers in particular, as promiscuous and careless. While the context of her everyday life with HIV has been shaped by her experiences with sexual violence and stigma, it has also been informed by her negotiation of degrees of visibility and invisibility within the spaces of the state, international agencies, and many HIV-related NGOs throughout Jamaica.

Asserting the need to expand current HIV prevention work in order to appropriately address the current landscape of HIV/AIDS, Dr. Nicola Skyers, the leader of Jamaica's NHP at the time, emphasized the need to address the "growing feminization of the epidemic" and to extend the exclusive focus of HIV interventions on traditional "at-risk populations" such as "MSM" and sex workers and toward the inclusion of women, youth, and other groups in the general population.[31] Like Star, many participants in EFL emphasized the need to amplify the voices of HIV+ young women in the national and regional responses.

Star's comment responded not only to the exclusion of youth and women in general, and young women in particular but also to the overriding presence of masculinist approaches to HIV prevention and care. Caribbean scholars have noted that this approach derives from the notorious use of the "male marginalization" theory, which often centered the "crisis" of Caribbean men and masculinity to bolster opposition to women's sexual and reproductive rights (Miller 1987). Such public debates and policy, as noted by Peggy Antrobus, focused on the "perceived link between the 'underachievement' of Caribbean males in the education system and advances in the status of women as a major contributory factor" (Antrobus 2005).[32] Extending these critiques of the male marginalization thesis, I use these case studies to insert the thoughts and experiences of Black Caribbean women into these constructions of racialized masculinity and sexuality as I shift attention to power dynamics in crisis narratives. In doing so, I posit that women's articulation of their embodied experiences of illness and marginalization enables them to simultaneously subvert both gendered inequities and erasures while mobilizing their bodies and voices on a broader scale to claim access to resources within public and private spaces of (mis)recognition.

Embodied knowledge is one of the practical results and political strategies of the interdependent relationships cultivated among HIV+ Black Caribbean women. I refer to embodied knowledge as the consciousness that emerges as women come to know and understand their bodies and sexualities through the relational and conflicting nature of the interplay of gender, race, colorism, sexuality, and illness in their everyday lives.[33] The intimate connections women develop in psychosocial support groups and the spaces of EFL extend to other private and public spaces frequented by high-level decision makers. Women learned about their bodies and reflected on the nature of their involvement in intimate relationships with romantic partners, family members, and children. They also learned how to use their knowledge of sexuality, health, and rights and their women-centered networks to resist the discrimination of some medical professionals who often imposed moral values about sexuality as well as to contest the research of public health practitioners who possessed the authority to support priority areas.

CONCLUSION

Donna, Tora, and Star attribute their mobilization around HIV with their own differential knowledge as HIV+, women, mothers, and as community leaders. It was precisely this knowledge that empowered young black Jamaican women around concerns beyond mere survival and medication adherence toward both prolonging and improving their quality of life, cultivating intergenerational bonds, and using the resources of EFL to combat gender inequality and their lack of political representation. The significance of women-centered networks of Caribbean women is no new discovery. Scholars have long theorized the intimacies that Caribbean women have cultivated and contested.[34] For example, Omise'eke Natasha Tinsley notes the significance of imaginative work in telling meaningful stories of black womanhood and sexuality. By foregrounding Barbara Christian's caution against "the race for theory" in her analysis of nonnormative and racialized people in the shipbuilding industry during World War II California, Tinsley offers creative methods and theoretical possibilities for theorizing narratives of Black women's freedom and erotic life beyond the official discourses that silence the telling of complex stories of gender, desire, and personhood in the African diaspora.[35] Given the range of quotidian intimacies, bodies, and self-refashioning among HIV+ women that exist beyond official documentation, Tinsley's question remains pertinent for this discussion of Black Caribbean women and the Black AIDS pandemic: "What else can Black women desire besides what the archive documents?" (Allen and Tinsley 2012, 251). The voices and experiences of young Jamaican women reveal that they can desire care, belonging, and solidarity. They uncover how these desires are rooted in the shared experiences of differently situated women who are invested in new kinds of community-building structures and embodied realities that counter the trope of HIV/AIDS containment and Black female pathology. These possibilities reveal the ways Caribbean women have connected their illness experiences to both legible and illegible identities as mothers, survivors, sexual subjects, and political actors in order to mobilize around the practical needs and strategic interests of themselves and their peers.

In conclusion, I ask: If the always healthy, always productive, and always resistant Black subject remains a prioritized figure in Black studies, then how do marginalized Black Caribbean women living with HIV matter to projects of Black sexual politics and Black liberation? Black Caribbean women challenge the portrayal of "non-American" subjects as undifferentiated and heteronormative while clarifying the need to identify new subjects and new sites of analyses about race, gender, sexuality, and health. In "Punks, Bulldaggers, and Welfare Queens: The Radical Potential of Queer Politics?", Cathy Cohen (1997) offers an invitation to think about queer heterosexuals beyond the norms of queer politics that have often served to reinforce simple dichotomies "between heterosexual and everything 'queer,'" subsuming differences of race, class, and gender.[36] Young HIV+ women in Jamaica are queered in relation to the colonial racialized and patriarchal terms which frame Black women as abject sexual subjects in a broader context of deteriorating material realities shaped by global health agencies and public health institutions that condemn their bodies, sexual choices, reproductive capacities, gendered performances, and modes of political participation. Thus, these women challenge the dichotomy that often exists between heterosexual and queer by using their voices and embodied political practices to intervene in the centrality of specific racialized (lighter-skinned) and classed (middle class and upper elites) bodies in official Jamaican discourses and public health campaigns as well as to contest the omnipresence of the (white) gay male body in dominant HIV/AIDS research and movements.[37] As they leverage these varied degrees of power, they undermine the coherence of queer and its relationship to a specific sexual identity or behavior because of the fluid connections they make between their sexual desires and practices coupled with their stigmatized embodiment. Their intersectional subject positions render more expansive readings of queerness, Black female sexuality, and HIV/AIDS because they signify resistances that originate from and in more shared experiences of racialized sexual and nonsexual marginalization and oppression.

Within this space of tension, possibility, and ambiguity are opportunities to expand our political and scholarly pursuits toward a more radically liberatory Black sexual politics, racialized gendered embodiment, and transnational responses to HIV/AIDS. We know far less about young HIV+ Black women as political actors and sexual subjects than we do about them as medical objects. Through my conversations and interactions with women like Donna, Tora, and Star within and beyond the spaces of EFL, I began to understand how their women-centered networks of care and holistic health within constricted social and institutional spaces provide a foundation for new expressions of Black erotic life and social intimacies. Given the scant literature on the pandemic among Black women in general, and Caribbean women in particular, and the lack of knowledge of their cultural work and intimate lives, this ethnographic study of young HIV+ Black Jamaican women in Kingston provides an appropriate basis from which to forge dialogues across (inter)disciplines, geographic locations, and cultural contexts as well as among activists, practitioners, and researchers. Grounding these dialogues in Black women's lives and cultural knowledge challenges current hegemonic HIV/AIDS discourses by revealing how differently located women make meaning as they shoulder the disproportionate burdens to manage illness and its uneven impacts on their communities. Furthermore, this chapter emphasizes the need for "positive living" programs to not only address the medical and physiological symptoms of illness but to also prioritize the psychic, emotional, and social impacts that undermine the possibilities of well-being, community care, and political organizing of people living with and impacted by HIV/AIDS. The holistic claims of women for political recognition, connection, and psychosocial care further illuminate the racial, gender, class, and geopolitical dynamics in the HIV apparatus, which challenges both the quantification of progress in the "end of HIV/AIDS" discourses and the tendency of "end of HIV/AIDS" discourses to compartmentalize women's lives in risk categories and medical subjects.

NOTES

1. This chapter was previously published in Jolly, Jallicia. "From 'at Risk' to Interdependent: The Erotic Life Worlds of HIV+ Jamaican Women." *Souls* 21, no. 2–3 (2019): 107–131.

2. I have translated to Standard American English from Jamaican Creole English, a creole language with West African and British English influences, in order to communicate the participants' ideas and opinions. Jamaican Creole English is also known as "patwah," a term which scholars note provides a characteristically Caribbean linguistic reframing to describe a creole language and not a dialect that is often viewed as substandard.

3. These names are pseudonyms. While I originally designed this study to be anonymous and confidential out of my desire to protect the privacy of the individuals and the organizations, some EFL participants wanted to be identified given the lack of documentation of Black women-centered HIV organizing. The project thus became one in which individuals and organizations could decide if and how they were to be identified in this study.

4. Jacqui Alexander's use of the "transnational" is instructive here: it grounds "historically intransigent colonial relationship[s], in which a previously scripted colonial cartography of ownership, production, consumption, and distribution all conform to a 'First World/Third World' division" (1998: 294). In this project, I use this framework to illustrate how women's political engagements with HIV interventions on the ground highlight the ongoing battles of differently located subjects to redefine and transform race-, gender-, and class-based inequities and women's exclusion in the HIV/AIDS movements. The recent scholarship of scholars such as Roderick Ferguson (2004), Rinaldo Walcott (2005, 2013), Michelle Wright and Antje Schuhmann (2007), Jafari Allen (2012), and Lyndon Gill (2018) who have engaged Black, queer, and diaspora simultaneously has broadened the geographic and thematic scopes of studies of Blackness and sexuality. I rely on Jafari Allen's use of Black queer diaspora as "a caution, a theory, and (most centrally) *a work*" that pushes the territories of queer theory and Black queer studies in different sites and forms by simultaneously deepening connections between scholarship and critical engagements with political organizing "in the context of various shifts in Empire(s) and affiliations" (Allen 2012: 214, 237).

5. I consider EFL a "framing institution," which Celeste Watkins-Hayes describes as "agents that help women revise their personal frameworks and directly challenge the societal narratives within which they initially frame the diagnosis" (2011: 2028). I similarly foreground the links Berger makes between identity, resources, and participation in her ethnographic exploration of how marginalization constrains Black

and Latina women's access to resources and services, ultimately shaping their health trajectories and political participation. See Celeste Watkins-Hayes, LaShawnDa Pittman-Gay, and Jean Beaman (2012) and Michele Tracy Berger (1998).

6. I join other critical HIV/AIDS researchers who have resisted the framing of HIV/AIDS as a "chronic condition." While mainstream narratives emphasize the transition of HIV from an inevitable "death sentence" to a "chronic condition" globally, Afro-diasporic people's social and political realities disrupt these linear notions of progress that often circulate in resourced countries such as the United States. Thus, the ongoing narratives that emphasize the path to the "End of AIDS" fail to align with the current trajectory of the epidemic and its subsequent racial, gendered, and classed dimensions, particularly in the lives of the multiply marginalized. Given that "the age of treatment" still does not include many people in these countries in the "Global South," it is crucial to note, as Eileen Moyer notes, that this period "is bounded less by time than it is by economics and geopolitics" (2015: 261).

7. UNAIDS, "Fast-Track strategy to end the AIDS epidemic by 2030" https://www.unaids.org/en/resources/campaigns/World-AIDS-Day-Report-2014 (accessed November 2015).

8. Black feminist scholarship and artistry has long engaged the dimensions of Black women's intimate lives. Some courageous visionaries include Toni Cade Bambara, Audre Lorde, Alice Walker, Faith Ringgold, June Jordan, and Ntozake Shange. Within a Jamaican context, these include Honor Ford Smith and Sistren Theatre Collective, Yanique Hume, Ebony Patterson, and Edna Madley. For more information on Black and Caribbean feminist artistry and scholarship, see Uri McMillan (2015), Davis et al. (2017), Smith (2010).

9. I echo the calls of previous scholars who caution against using labels of sexuality on non-European people in contexts such as the Caribbean and Latin America. In particular, Gloria Wekker cautions against adopting Western labels of sexual constructions that homogenize cultures while privileging certain social experiences (2007: 191, 213, 224). For more elaborate discussions about cultural constructions of same-sex sexuality as well as the uses of "MSM" in the social science literature, see Blackwood (1986), Wekker (2006), Padilla (2007), Mitchell (2016).

10. Lyndon Gill describes the erotic in three parts as "various formal and informal power hierarchies (the political), sexual as well as non-sexual intimacy (the sensual), and sacred metaphysics (the spiritual)" (2012: 10). Gill conceptualizes the "erotic subjectivity" as encompassing a "political attentiveness and spiritual consciousness" that is a "tripartite political-sensual-spiritual awareness makes possible and desirable a more broadly and deeply conceived articulation of love" (2012: 280).

11. I rely on Audre Lorde's definition of the erotic as "a resource within reach of us that lies in a deeply female and spiritual plane, firmly rooted in the power of our unexpressed and unrecognized feeling" (Lorde [1978] (1984), 53). My understanding of the erotic is also heavily informed by Lyndon Gill's discussion of a praxis of survival that is rooted in an 'interlinked spiritual-sensual-political (erotic) subjectivity' which he uses to describe the intimate connections among queer Caribbean subjects who face multiple oppressions. Recent work in Caribbean Studies has built upon

Lorde's conception of the erotics to elucidate the dynamics among quotidian life, political possibilities, subjectivities, and black queerness throughout the Caribbean and the African diaspora. See Audre Lorde (1984), Gill (2018, 2012), King (2014), Sheller (2012), Allen (2011), Tinsley (2010).

12. I consider how women insist on sexual agency while resisting heteronormativity. For more discussion about expansive models of complex black subjectivities that embrace a resistant insistence on pleasure, see Horton-Stallings (2015).

13. In recent years, Black and Caribbean feminist scholarship of sexuality by scholars such as Lyndon Gill (2018), Jennifer Nash (2014), Rosamond King (2014), Marlon Bailey (2013), Mireille Miller-Young (2013), Mimi Sheller (2012), LaMonda Horton-Stallings (2007), and Gloria Wekker (2006) has departed from ideological, political, and cultural investments in sexual morality and respectability in favor of elucidating more diverse sexual realities of nonnormative Black subjects.

14. For an imaginative conversation on locating a political agency and sexual universe that escapes colonial archival record and official documentation of governments, institutions, and scholars, see Sheller (2012).

15. Recent scholarship on gender, sexuality, and political movements in the Caribbean has noted the transnational politics of organizing strategies. Noteworthy is Matthew Chin's discussion of "gaydren" as a transnational political practice reflected in the cultural work of Jamaican activists who contest normative configurations of gay and *bredren* while transforming rigid political discourses around sexual politics (2019).

16. I embrace the insights of scholars such as Lyndon Gill, Marlon Bailey, and Michelle Tracey Berger who center ethnography in their study of HIV/AIDS in Black communities. Additionally, feminist ethnography's emphasis on subaltern ways of knowing and reflexivity allows for more ethical and culturally informed observations and interpretations of interactions and conversations in naturally occurring situations. For more on reflexivity and feminist ethnography, see Kamala Visweswaran (1994) and Lather (2001). For further discussions on how gender, sexuality, illness, and marginalization shape lived experiences, see Gill (2018), Bailey (2013), and Berger (1998).

17. Jamaica became one of the four countries in Latin America and the Caribbean in 2005 named "champion countries" by the United Nations Global Fund for HIV/AIDS, for its work to protect against and educate children about the epidemic. For more information on the initial stages of the epidemic, see Olukoga (2004).

18. Ministry of Health, "HIV Epidemiological Profile 2015, Facts & Figures," last modified May 4, 2017, accessed November 2017, https://www.moh.gov.jm/data/hiv-epidemiological-profile-2015-facts-figures/; UNAIDS Global AIDS Response Progress Report, "Jamaica Country Progress Report, March 31, 2014," accessed November 2017, https://www.unaids. org/sites/default/files/country/documents/JAMnarrativereport2014.pdf.

19. Ibid.

20. See Gina Ulysse's incisive analysis of how the socioeconomic practices and self-making strategies contest the traditional binaries of lady/woman and uptown/downtown that are rooted in racial and gender hierarchies that are color-coded (2007).

21. Jamaica has the third largest population of people living with HIV/AIDS in the Caribbean, after the Dominican Republic and Haiti (MOH 2001). Haitians became the only national group marked as at risk for AIDS by the Center for Disease Control (the United States' official governing institution of public health) in the early 1980s. A *New York Times* article chronicled the international response (see Altman 1983).

22. In contrast to the initial years of the AIDS epidemic in the United States, where the behavioral categories of "MSM," injecting drug users, and hemophiliacs emerged as categories of "risk" as defined by surveillance bodies, in Jamaica the initial categories were both occupationally and behaviorally driven, with migrant workers, commercial sex workers, out-of-school youth, MSM, and the generalized population identified as "risk groups." During the second decade as the epidemic became more generalized and mother-to-child transmission rates increased alongside growing teenage pregnancy rates, some attention to Jamaica's epidemic turned to the broader concern of girls and young women's sexual vulnerability and the prevention of mother-to-child transmission of HIV. See Figueroa (2014).

23. By making a distinction between identity and praxis in the approach to sexuality, Kamala Kempadoo moves us beyond the exclusive focus on sexual behavior and sexuality as a primary basis for social identification, which creates more complete understandings of the sexual arrangements in the region and in broader African diasporic social life.

24. In recent years, HIV/AIDS researchers have increasingly used interdisciplinary frameworks rooted in the culturally specific realities of Caribbean youth to unpack rigid measures of risk and vulnerability. Noteworthy is Orlando Harris's discussion of the sociostructural factors that influence the sexual decision making among young Jamaican MSM who engaged in transactional sex as a result of homelessness, family neglect, or limited financial resources. See Harris (2019: 883–897).

25. "Jamaica Gets Millions in HIV/AIDS Funding," Ministry of Health, National HIV/STI Program, last modified July 15, 2015, http://moh.gov.jm/jamaica-gets-millions-in-hiv-funding/.

26. This is not to say that local Caribbean organizations do not find creative and strategic ways to develop and implement their own agendas while navigating these controlling forces. As noted by queer Caribbean feminists Rosamond King and Angelique Nixon in their discussion of the relationship between Caribbean feminism, feminist practice, and sexuality studies, they argue that it is through "local scholarly and non-scholarly knowledges, community-organizing, and embodied theories that we can transform the limited discourses around sex and sexuality for Caribbean people generally" (2013: 11).

27. The parishes of Kingston and St. James are key sites to investigate the cultural politics of HIV/AIDS. St. James remains the parish with a significant tourism-based economy and the highest level of cumulative number of reported HIV cases since the start of the epidemic in the 1980s (MOH 2010). Kingston is also the site for various social welfare agencies and HIV/AIDS NGOs, many of which provide care and advocacy for the rights of children, women, and their families, as well as the disabled and sexual minorities such as lesbians, gay men, and transgender people. Both Montego

Bay and Kingston share deep and highly visible inequalities between the poor, working poor, and elites, as well as grave social and economic inequalities.

28. I rely on Juana Maria Rodriguez's definition of interdependence as a value and commitment that is "built on mutual respect and consideration, absent coercion, in the search for mutual pleasure, in the search for other sexual futures" (Rodriguez 2015: 96).

29. In 2016, Mentor Moms usually received a monthly stipend of JD 30,000 (USD 250) for their provision of services. Mentee Moms received JD 1,500–3,000 (USD 12.50–25) for their attendance at each workshop and additional meetings as well as occasional care packages. While having a steady income, Mentor Moms often noted that the costs of childcare, school fees, housing, food, and additional work-related costs of transportation to and from outreach events make it challenging to meet all of their monthly expenses.

30. The 25th Annual Review and Planning Retreat conference gathered over 200 health care providers, government officials, civil society organization leaders, and international donors to discuss the trajectory of the HIV epidemic in Jamaican, review previous interventions, and develop new strategies for moving forward. I served as a note-taker for the duration of the conference.

31. I agree with critiques that note the limitation of the categories "MSM" and "female sex workers" which conflate sexual practices with sexual orientation and occupation, ignoring the spectrum of intimate exchanges that shape sexual relationships and encounters. According to Mark Padilla, this approach frames bisexual behavior as incidental and sporadic, and the men who "deviate" from hegemonic heterosexuality as culpable in the spread of the disease to the rest of the population (2007). See also Blackwood (1986) and Mitchell (2016).

32. Similarly, Eudine Barriteau encourages scholars and practitioners to address the ways the assumed relative disadvantage of men neglects a complete analysis of the formal and informal state action, juridical decisions, gender inequities, and lived experiences that shape differential access to and distribution of material resources and nonmaterial resources of status, power, and privilege among women and men. For more discussions about gender inequality, Caribbean feminisms, and identity development in the region, see Barriteau (2001) and Mohammed (1998).

33. I developed my understanding of embodied knowledge to further highlight how HIV+ Black women's experiences and perspectives intervene in the conventional theorizing of racial, gender, and sexual politics. I locate this analysis in the thought of Norma Alarc´on, Gloria Anzaldu´a, Chela Sandoval, Deborah King, and Patricia Hill Collins who have challenged claims of universality in terms of gender and race by emphasizing consciousness as a site of multiple voicings and the urgency of a multivalent praxis. This understanding moves beyond the additive approaches to conceptualizing oppression that subsumes one type of oppression under another. In rejecting this approach, Black and women of color feminist scholars have developed alternative models that have considered how intersecting oppressions have coalesced in their lives. See Anzaldu´a (1987), King (1988), Collins (2008), Sandoval (1991).

34. Caribbean women writers such as Jamaica Kincaid, Maryse Conde, and Paule Marshall have developed multifaceted links that bind women to each other

and to their children. They have been foundational in demonstrating how the centrality of motherhood and femininity in these networks as loci of female social identity in both home and host countries drives expressions and understandings of belonging and home. For example, Audre Lorde's women-centered networks in *Zami* are sources and resources that lead her "home" to her domestic past in the Caribbean community of Harlem and "home" to Grenada, which guides her engagements with a multiplicity of histories, communities, and selves in her work. See Lorde (1982).

35. In her incisive article, "The Race for Theory," Barbara Christian challenged the increasing domination of African American literary study by those who were primarily interested in theory rather than in writers and their work. Her critique of the continual race for theory, a race that sometimes leaves the literature itself in the dust, provides a starting point for Black women writers theorizing with their literature and using their lived experiences. See Christian (1987).

36. Cohen's (1997) article along with Jos´e Esteban Muñoz's *Disidentifications* (1999) and Roderick Ferguson's *Aberrations in Black* (2004) made evident how queer theory, gay and lesbian studies, and the history of sexuality excluded and rendered obsolete a critical intersectional analysis on race. Recent works by Ferguson (2012), Hong and Ferguson (2011), and Juana Maria Rodriguez (2014) have extended these critiques of racialized sexuality and heteronormativity.

37. I recognize the contributions of gay male activists in the early years of the pandemic in the United States and the Caribbean, which helped expand AIDS activism and develop an infrastructure and social services that now support HIV/AIDS. I also heed the calls of feminist HIV researchers to elevate the elided histories and labor of women of color and lesbians who cared for each other and the living and dying among them. For more information on these gendered and racialized erasures and the impacts of this early activism, refer to Watkins-Hayes (2019) and Schulman (1994).

REFERENCES

Alexander, M. Jacqui. 1994. "Not Just (Any) Body Can Be a Citizen: The Politics of Law, Sexuality and Postcoloniality in Trinidad and Tobago and the Bahamas." *Feminist Review*, no. 48: 5–23. https://doi.org/10.2307/1395166.

Alexander, M. Jacqui and Lisa Albrecht, eds. 1998. *The Third Wave: Feminist Perspectives on Racism*. New York: Kitchen Table: Women of Color Press.

Allen, Jafari S. 2011. *iVenceremos?: The Erotics of Black Self-Making in Cuba*. Durham NC: Duke University Press.

Allen, Jafari S. 2012. "Black/Queer/Diaspora at the Current Conjuncture." *GLQ: A Journal of Lesbian and Gay Studies* 18, no. 2: 211–48.

Allen, Jafari S., and Omise'eke Natasha Tinsley. 2012. "A Conversation 'Overflowing with Memory'On Omise'eke Natasha Tinsley's 'Water, Shoulders, Into the Black Pacific.'" *GLQ: A Journal of Lesbian and Gay Studies* 18, no. 2–3: 249–62. https://doi.org/10.1215/10642684-1472881.

Altman, Lawrence K. 1983. Debate Grows on U.S. Listing of Haitians in AIDS Category." *New York Times*, July 31 1983. https://www.nytimes.com/1983/07/31/us/ debate-grows-on-us-listing-of-haitians-in-aids-category.html.
Antrobus, Peggy. 2005. "Critiquing the MDGs from a Caribbean Perspective 1." *Gender & Development* 13, no. 1: 94–104. https://doi.org/10.1080/13552070512331332280.
Anzaldu´a, Gloria. 1987. *Borderlands/La frontera: The New Mestiza.* San Francisco: Spinsters/Aunt Lute.
Bailey, M. 2013. *Butch Queens Up in Pumps: Gender, Performance, and Ballroom Culture in Detroit.* Ann Arbor: University of Michigan Press.
Bailey, Marlon M. 2009. "Performance as Intravention: Ballroom Culture and the Politics of HIV/AIDS in Detroit." *Souls: A Critical Journal of Black Politics, Culture, and Society* 11, no. 3: 253–74.
Barriteau, Eudine. 2001. *The Political Economy of Gender in the Twentieth-Century Caribbean.* New York: Palgrave Macmillan.
Berger, Michele Tracy. 2010. *Workable Sisterhood: The Political Journey of Stigmatized Women with HIV/AIDS*. Princeton, N.J.: Princeton University Press.
Blackwood, Evelyn. 1986. "Reading Sexualities across Cultures: Anthropology and Theories of Sexuality." *Gender and Society* 19, no. 2: 69–92.
Chin, Matthew. 2019. "Constructing 'Gaydren': The Transnational Politics of Same-Sex Desire in 1970s and 1980s Jamaica." *SmallAxe* 2, no. 2: 17–33.
Christian, Barbara. 1987. "The Race for Theory." *Cultural Critique* no. 6: 51–63. https://doi.org/10.2307/1354255.
Cohen, Cathy J. 1999. *The Boundaries of Blackness: AIDS and the Breakdown of Black Politics*. Chicago: University of Chicago Press.
Cohen, Cathy J. 1997. "Punks, Bulldaggers, and Welfare Queens: The Radical Potential of Queer Politics?" *GLQ: A Journal of Lesbian and Gay Studies* 3, no. 4: 437–65. https://doi.org/10.1215/10642684-3-4-437.
Collins, Patricia Hill. 2008. *Black Feminist Thought: Knowledge, Consciousness, and the Politics of Empowerment.* New York: Routledge.
Collins, Patricia Hill. 2004. *Black Sexual Politics : African Americans, Gender, and the New Racism.* New York: Routledge.
Davis, Annalee, Joscelyn Gardner, Erica Moiah James, and Jerry Philogene. 2017. "Introduction: Art as Caribbean Feminist Practice." *Small Axe: A Caribbean Journal of Criticism* 21, no. 1: 34–42. https://doi.org/10.1215/07990537-3844046.
Farmer, Paul. 2004. "An Anthropology of Structural Violence." *Current Anthropology* 45, no. 3: 305–25. https://doi.org/10.1086/382250.
Ferguson, Roderick A. 2004. *Aberrations in Black: Toward a Queer of Color Critique*. Minneapolis: University of Minnesota Press.
Ferguson, Roderick. A. 2012. *The Reorder of Things: The University and its Pedagogies of Minority Difference*. Minneapolis. University of Minnesota Press.
Figueroa, J. Peter. 2014. "Review of HIV in the Caribbean: Significant Progress and Outstanding Challenges." *Current HIV/AIDS Reports* 11: 158–167. https://doi.org /10.1007/ s11904-014-0199-7.

Gill, Lyndon K. 2012. "Chatting Back an Epidemic: Caribbean Gay Men, HIV/AIDS, and the Uses of Erotic Subjectivity." *GLQ: A Journal of Lesbian and Gay Studies* 8, no. 2–3: 277–95. https://doi.org/10.1215/10642684-1472899.

Gill, Lyndon. 2018. *Erotic Islands: Art and Activism in the Queer Caribbean*. Duke University Press.Hong, Grace and Roderick Ferguson. 2011. *Strange Affinities: The Gender and Sexual Politics of Comparative Racialization*. Durham: Duke University Press.

Horton-Stallings, Lamonda. 2015. *Funk the Erotic: Transaesthetics and Black Sexual Cultures*. Urbana-Champaign: University of Illinois Press.

Kempadoo, Kamala. 2009. "Caribbean Sexuality: Mapping the Field." *Caribbean Review of Gender Studies*, no. 3: 1–24. https://sta.uwi.edu/crgs/november2009/

King, Deborah. 1988. "Multiple Jeopardy, Multiple Consciousness: The Context of a Black Feminist Ideology." *Signs* 14, no. 1: 42–72.

King, Rosamond. 2014. *Island Bodies: Transgressive Sexualities in the Caribbean Imagination*. Miami: University of Florida.

LaBennett, Oneka. 2011. *She's Mad Real: Popular Culture and West Indian Girls in Brooklyn*. New York: NYU Press.

Lather, Patti. 2001. "Postbook: Working the Ruins of Feminist Ethnography." *Signs* 27, no. 1: 199–227.

Lorde, Audre. 1984. *Sister Outsider: Essays and Speeches. Trumansburg*. New York: Crossing Press.

Lorde, Audre. 1982. *A New Spelling of My Name*. Freedom, CA: The Crossing Press.

McMillan, Uri. 2015. *Embodied Avatars: Genealogies of Black Feminist Art and Performance*. New York: NYU Press.

Miller, Errol. 1987. *Marginalization of the Black Male*. Mona, Jamaica: Institute of Social and Economic Research, University of the West Indies.

Miller-Young, Mireille. 2014. *A Taste for Brown Sugar: Black Women in Pornography*. Durham, NC: Duke University Press Books.

Ministry of Health. 2017. "HIV Epidemiological Profile 2015, Facts & Figures." Accessed November 2017. https://www.moh.gov.jm/data/hiv-epidemiological- profile-2015-facts-figures/.

Ministry of Health. 2015. "Jamaica Gets Millions in HIV/AIDS Funding." National HIV/STI Program. Accessed November 2015. http://moh.gov.jm/jamaica-gets-millions-in-hiv-funding/.

Mitchell, Gregory. 2016. *Tourist Attractions: Performing Race and Masculinity in Brazil's Sexual Economy*. Chicago: University of Chicago Press.

Mohammed, Patricia. 1998. *Rethinking Caribbean Difference*. Psychology Press.

Moyer, Eileen. 2015. "The Anthropology of Life After AIDS: Epistemological Continuities in the Age of Antiretroviral Treatment." *Annual Review of Anthropology* 44, no. 1: 259–75.https://doi.org/10.1146/annurev-anthro-102214-014235.

Muñoz, José Esteban. 1999. *Disidentifications: Queers of Color and the Performance of Politics*. Minneapolis, MN: University of Minnesota Press.

Nash, Jennifer. 2019. *Black Feminism Reimagined: After Intersectionality*. Durham, NC: Duke University Press.

Nixon, Angelique and Rosamond King. 2013. "Embodied Theories: Local Knowledge(s), Community Organizing, and Feminist Methodologies in Caribbean Sexuality Studies." *Caribbean Review of Gender Studies* no. 7, 1–15. https://issuu.com/igdssau/docs/crgs_issue7_december2013.

Olukoga, Idowu A. 2004. "Epidemiologic Trends of HIV/AIDS in Jamaica." *Pan American Journal of Public Health* 15, no. 5: 358–63.

Orlando Harris. 2019. "Survival now versus survival later: immediate and delayed HIV risk assessment among young Jamaican men who have transactional sex with men." *Culture, Health & Sexuality* 21, no. 8: 883–97.

Padilla, Mark. 2007. *Caribbean Pleasure Industry: Tourism, Sexuality and AIDS in the Dominican Republic.* Chicago: University of Chicago Press.

Parikh, Shanti A. 2007. "The Political Economy of Marriage and HIV: The ABC Approach, 'Safe' Infidelity, and Managing Moral Risk in Uganda." *American Journal of Public Health* 97, no. 7: 1198–208. https://doi.org/10.2105/AJPH.2006.088682.

Parker, Richard. 2001. "Sexuality, Culture, and Power in HIV/AIDS Research." *Annual Review of Anthropology* 30: 163–79. https://doi.org/10.1146/annurev.anthro.30.1.163.

Rodríguez, Juana María. 2014. *Sexual Futures, Queer Gestures, and Other Latina Longings*. New York: NYU Press.

Sandoval, Chela. 1991. "U.S. Third World Feminism: The Theory and Method of Oppositional Consciousness in the Postmodern World." *Genders* no. 10: 1–24.

Schulman, Sarah. 1994. *My American History: Lesbian and Gay Life during the Reagan/Bush Years*. New York: Routledge,.

Sheller, Mimi. 2012. *Citizenship from Below: Erotic agency and Caribbean Freedom.* Durham, NC: Duke University Press.

Smith, Karina. 2010. "Struggling to Cross the Race and Class Divide: Sistren's Theatrical and Organizational Model of Collectivity." *Theatre Research International* 36, no. 2: 64–78.

Springer, Kimberly. 2005. *Living for the Revolution: Black Feminist Organizations, 1968–1980*. Durham, NC: Duke University Press.

Tinsley, Omise'eke Natasha. 2008. "Black Atlantic, Queer Altantic: Queer Imaginings of the Middle Passage." *GLQ: A Journal of Lesbian and Gay Studies* 14, no. 2–3: 191–215. https://doi.org/10.1215/10642684-2007-030.

Tinsley, Omise'eke Natasha. 2012. "Extract from 'Water, Shoulders, Into the Black Pacific.'" *GLQ: A Journal of Lesbian and Gay Studies* 18, no. 2–3: 263–76. https://doi.org/10.1215/10642684-1472890.

Tinsley, Omise'eke Natasha. 2010. *Thiefing Sugar: Eroticism between Women in Caribbean Literature*. Durham, NC: Duke University Press.

Ulysse, Gina A. 2007. *Downtown Ladies: Informal Commercial Importers, a Haitian Anthropologist and Self-Making in Jamaica*. University of Chicago Press.

UNAIDS. 2015. "Fast-Track strategy to end the AIDS epidemic by 2030." Accessed November 2015.https://www.unaids.org/en/resources/campaigns/World-AIDS-Day-Report-2014.

UNAIDS. 2017. Global AIDS Response Progress Report. "Jamaica Country Progress Report March 31, 2014." Accessed November 2017, https://www.unaids.org/sites/default/files/country/ documents/JAMnarrativereport2014.pdf.

Visweswaran, Kamala. 1994. *Fictions of Feminist Ethnography*. University of Minnesota Press.

Walcott, Rinaldo. 2013. "Black Queer Studies, Freedom, and Other Human Possibilities." In *Understanding Blackness through Performance: Contemporary Arts and the Representation of Identity*, edited by Anne Crémieux, Xavier Lemoine, and Jean-Paul Rocchi, 143–57. New York: Palgrave Macmillan US.

Walcott, Rinaldo. 2005. "Outside in Black Studies: Reading from a Queer Place in the Diaspora." In *Black Queer Studies: A Critical Anthology*, edited by Johnson, E. Patrick, and Mae G. Henderson, 90–105. Durham, NC: Duke University Press Books.

Watkins-Hayes, Celeste. 2008. "The Social and Economic Context of Black Women Living with HIV/AIDS in the US: Implications for Research." In *Sex, Power, and Taboo: Gender and HIV in the Caribbean and Beyond*, edited by Rhoda Reddock, Sandra Reid, Dianne Douglas, and Dorothy Roberts, 33–66. Kingston, Jamaica: Ian Randle Publishers.

Watkins-Hayes, Celeste. 2019. *Remaking a Life: How Women Living with HIV/AIDS Confront Inequality*. Berkeley: University of California Press.

Watkins-Hayes, Celeste, LaShawnDa Pittman-Gay, and Jean Beaman. 2012. "'Dying from' to 'Living with': Framing Institutions and the Coping Processes of African American Women Living with HIV/AIDS." *Social Science & Medicine* 74, no. 12: 2028–36.

Wekker, Gloria. 2006. *The Politics of Passion: Women's Sexual Culture in the Afro-Surinamese Diaspora*. New York: Columbia University Press.

White, Ruth C., and Robert Carr. 2005, "Homosexuality and HIV/AIDS Stigma in Jamaica." *Culture, Health & Sexuality* 7, no. 4: 347–59. https://doi.org/10.1080/13691050500100799.

Whiteside, Alan. 2008. *HIV/AIDS: A Very Short Introduction*. Oxford: Oxford University Press.

Wright, Michelle M. and Ante Schuhmann. 2007. *Blackness and Sexualities*. Berlin: LIT Verlag.

Chapter 9

Life beyond Survival

HIV+ Men on ART Treatment Who Consume Alcohol in Urban India

Stephen L. Schensul

This chapter examines the adaptations and challenges of HIV+ men treated in hospital-based antiretroviral therapy (ART) centers in greater Mumbai, India, who consume alcohol.[1] The chapter draws on qualitative and baseline quantitative data, collected as a part of the formative phase of a National Institute of Alcohol Abuse and Alcoholism (NIAAA) (2014–2020) research and intervention project focused on reducing alcohol use and increasing ART medication adherence in the greater Mumbai, India area. The objective of this formative research phase was to increase the acceptability and relevance of the subsequent stages of the project including the development and implementation of multilevel interventions and the quantitative measurement of intervention impact using a controlled experimental trial. These data indicate that while ART medication meets many of the physical challenges of HIV, the associated psychological, substance use, social and societal issues that accompany the disease remain mostly unaddressed with significant implications for its transformation from an infectious and life threatening to a chronic disease.

Antiretroviral medication has been deemed "a spectacular success" (Deeks et al. 2013), keeping people living with HIV (PLHIV) healthy, adding decades to longevity, and reducing the risk of transmission. Despite the lack of a protective vaccine, ART has created the hopeful expectation that by 2030, we will see "the end of AIDS" (Fauci and Folkers 2012). However, before we declare that we are on the road to the control and elimination of the disease, there are ongoing biomedical and societal problems that remain unaddressed or not fully addressed that compromise the care of PLHIV.

First, ART provides the capacity to "control," but not "cure." For the foreseeable future, individuals who acquire HIV must be on lifelong medication, since ART cannot fully restore immunological health. As a result, PLHIV treated with ART can frequently experience the biophysiological effects of toxic ART medications including inflammation-associated and/or immunodeficiency complications such as cardiovascular, kidney, and liver disease and cancer that can result in accelerated aging (Deeks et al. 2013). Our knowledge of these long-term physical effects of lifelong ART medication is still evolving (Sangaramoorthy 2018).

Engagement of PLHIV in the treatment cascade continues to be a problem. UNAIDS developed the HIV treatment cascade goal of 90% tested, 90% in treatment, and 90% with undetectable viral load (UNAIDS 2014). A 2016 review (Levi et al. 2016) found that in 69 countries, testing ranged from 87% (the Netherlands) to 11% (Yemen), treatment coverage ranged from 71% (Switzerland) to 3% (Afghanistan), and viral suppression was between 68% (Switzerland) and 7% (China). The United States, with 84% diagnosed, 61% entering care, but only 48% retained and 49% with undetectable viral load, falls well below these cascade goals. For India, 79% knew their HIV-positive status, 56% are in treatment, and 40–50% have an undetectable viral load: these rates are comparable to the United States (National AIDS Control Organization (NACO) 2017) but with a long way to go to achieve UNAIDS treatment cascade goals.

There has been a significant global reduction in new cases of HIV. Nonetheless, the global estimate of an annual 550,000 individuals with new infections, in combination with the need for lifetime treatment of current PLHIV, and the need to engage many who are not in treatment, puts an excessive burden on health care systems, particularly those in low- and middle-income countries (LMICs). The Government of India (GOI) through its lead agency, the NACO, rolled out free ART medication in 2004 and there are now close to 500 centers in all states. India has an estimated 88,000 new infections annually, combined with the extended longevity of the current 1.2 million patients requiring lifelong care and continuing efforts to reach the estimated 900,000 not in care. The GOI can therefore anticipate significant growth in future patient load at a time when most HIV treatment facilities have already far exceeded their capacity. Currently, ART centers in India and other LMICs are coping with increased crowding, limited staff and program resources, and abandoning specialized clinics to integrate HIV treatment into the general primary care system in an effort to reduce cost.

Insufficient adherence (<95%) by a significant subset of PLHIV to ART medication can contribute to first-line medication failure and detectable viral load. One of the key factors in nonadherence involves alcohol consumption. The research literature over the past decade consistently shows that alcohol consumption has a negative impact on the health status of PLHIV. These effects include reduced immunological function (Chawla & Ichhpujani 2011), nonadherence to ART medication (Kalichman et al., 2013), increased comorbidities (Mather et al., 2013), greater risky sexual behavior (Yadav 2014), and greater likelihood of dropping out of all components of the treatment cascade (Williams et al., 2019). Alcohol use among PLHIV is not an isolated behavior, but is associated with negative emotional states (Ha et al. 2018), internalized and external stigma, and associated concerns about disclosing HIV status (Stringer et al. 2019).

The continued societal stigmatization of HIV/AIDS, the structural issues related to the delivery of care, the reduction in resources for prevention and treatment, and the impact on PLHIV and their families suggest that effective medication is just one part of a comprehensive approach to the challenges and needs of PLHIV. Alcohol consumption adds another complicating dimension, bringing its own biophysiological, societal, and social issues. This chapter describes the adaptations of alcohol-consuming PLHIV as they cope with these multiple issues.

METHODOLOGY

The data for this chapter draws from an NIAAA/National Institutes of Health (NIH)-funded research, intervention, and evaluation project entitled "Alcohol and ART Adherence: Assessment, Intervention and Modeling in India" (2014–2020). The project was a collaboration of the Department of Public Health Sciences of University of Connecticut School of Medicine and the Institute for Community Research on the United States side and the Population Council, the ICRW, and the Network of Maharashtra People with HIV (NMP+) on the India side. With the help of NACO and its state and municipal subsidiaries, 5 of 13 ART centers in the greater Mumbai area were selected for inclusion in the study. An anonymous screener administered to 9,950 male PLHIV in the five ART centers awaiting treatment and medication pickup, established study eligibility in terms of age (21–65), length of time on ART medication (at least six months), and alcohol use (having consumed at least one drink of alcohol in the last 30 days). The final sample meeting these criteria included 55 PLHIV selected for in-depth interviews and 940 (188 in each center) agreeing to participate in the study and respond to baseline and follow-up surveys and viral load testing to assess intervention impact. This chapter utilizes the in-depth interviews, with support from the baseline survey data, to examine the lives of HIV+ men on ART treatment who consume alcohol and are dealing with the continuing issues of being HIV+ in the Indian societal, social, and familial context.

RESULTS

Demographic and HIV Status Characteristics

The mean age of the male PLHIV sample is 42.9 (SD = 8.35). The majority of the sample are migrants from the northern impoverished states, who are now long-term residents of greater Mumbai (mean = 24 years). Education and income show a bimodal distribution indicating that both lower and middle-income PLHIV take advantage of the availability of free ART medication provided by the government as compared with costly private care. Over 90% of the men are employed, an indicator that ART medication had contributed to their ability to keep working. PLHIV in this sample were diagnosed at a mean of 5.7 years ago and have been on ART medication for a mean of 4.7 years, well after the NACO rollout of free medication. At the time of the baseline interview, 10.2% (102) of the survey sample were single, never married and 89.8% (838) were ever married. Among the ever-married men, 77.7% (651) were married and living with their wives, 14.2% (119) were married and not living with their wives. Most of the wives not living with their husbands had returned to their natal families in their rural villages because of their positive HIV status or their husbands. Of the ever-married men, 8.1% (68) reported that their wives had died of whom, 60% were HIV+. Men in the survey sample reported that their wives had died, of whom 60% were HIV+, 53% were seronegative, and 5.3% in which their wives' status was unknown. Of those wives who were HIV+, 84.0% were on ART.

Among the PLHIV sample, 84.1% (783) reported that they were 100% ART adherent over the previous four days. Testing conducted by a lab contracted by project showed that 38.7% (314) had a detectable viral load (>20 copies per milliliter). CD4 testing conducted by the centers showed that 33.5% (310) had a count of 350 or less. Approximately 20% showed moderate to high problematic drinking, less than 90% adherence, and poor CD4 and viral load indicators of health status.

Transmission

Most men believed that they contracted HIV because of drinking alcohol with friends followed by having unprotected sex with sex workers. They describe in the in-depth interviews having *masti* (fun) with alcohol as a key component of these outings and a mutually supported, alcohol-fueled desire to have sex.

> We [friends] began drinking *desi daaru* [country brew] together and one day, we decided to go to the red light area. It was my first time to visit that place. I

feared at first but then I started to go for the sex again and again in different red light areas. (Age 38, 7 years of schooling, married for 14 years, 1 child)

I was 19 years old when we went to red light area. It was my first time to visit that place. I feared and then my friends gave me the support. And then we entered that house and lots of girls were standing there. I went with one girl for sex. Then I started to go for the sex again and again. I was enjoying my life with my friends. We went in the Ganesh festival. In that festival most of the sex workers come there for earning and there I paid one lady 200 rupees [approximately US$4.00] it was costly for me. Mostly I always used condoms but I don't know after drinking whether I used or not. I think for that reason I am suffering. When I was going for the sex, that time there was not any kind of compulsion to use of condom. (Age 40, 10 years of schooling, married for 19 years, 2 children)

Response to Diagnosis

Almost all the men interviewed experienced shock at the news of their HIV diagnosis. Reactions included self-blame, concern for their reputation and that of their families, and the reaction of their wives or their future marriageability.

I started to go with my friends for drinking and to the sex workers. I began to suffer from loose motion and fever and my father admitted me in government hospital. After one day then my family members and my relatives came to see me and came to know about my status. I was in trouble since my family has good reputation (*izzat)* in the village. They started ART treatment because my CD4 was too low. I feared my family members and neighbors. I was living in my bedroom only, I never go outside. My family members were not talking with me. Even my mother and father were also not talking with me. (Age 31, eight years of schooling, unmarried)

When I was 25 years my relatives arranged my marriage. They saw one girl and we met. I liked her and she also liked me. I was driving autorickshaw and earning very well then they fixed my marriage with that girl. I loved my wife and left going with friends for drinking and the red light area for the sex. After few months, I got good news from my wife, she was pregnant. Everyone was happy. Then my mother and she went to the hospital for the registration and a blood test. After two days she got the report of her HIV test and it was positive. Second day I went with her. They took my blood and I also got my HIV+ report. When my son completed 18 months, then they had done the HIV test and it was negative, thank God. When my son was three years old, that time my wife died. (Age 44, 7 years of education, 17 years of marriage, 1 child)

My wife, my mother, my son and I lived together. From wrong behavior [drinking and visiting sex workers] I was HIV+. It was my mistake and now she [wife] is no more. Now, I am living only for my son and my mother. I don't have any support from my relatives; they don't come here to meet us. I can't explain to my mother about my HIV status. She is aged now and how she will take this that I don't know. And I have fear of this situation; after her who will take care of my child. (Age 40, 5 years of education, 13 years of marriage, 1 child)

I always feel guilty. What I did? What this happened with me? I will lose my business if people know about my status. Then how they will think about me and my reputation? They always think negatively. (Age 39, 14 years of education, 2 years of marriage, no children)

It is compulsory to drink and have sex. We contact on phone and bring two girls in lodge for full night in Rs. 2000/ from red light area and enjoy drink and sex. But once my friend became HIV+ and died we stopped those things. Another committed suicide, and a few of them left village after some time. (Age 29, seven years of schooling, unmarried)

Internal Stigma

For a subset of PLHIV, the feelings of self-blame or internalized stigma continued well beyond the immediate period after diagnosis, while for others the feelings of guilt diminished as they learned to manage their illness.

Some time I still get angry on myself. I always ask the question to myself, what I did. And how you will face to the society? But I knew this is happened because of me. I have guilt also. And sometimes I feel to finish myself. (Age 36, 12 years of education, never married)

I was diagnosed with HIV 4 years ago. I was alone. I suffered from mental trauma. I was having tension of my illness, that time I thought of committing suicide but I could not do that when I thought about my son. He would have become an orphan, so I thought of not spoiling my son's life because of my illness. I should live at least for him. These thoughts changed my opinion of ending my life. (Age 47, 12 years of education, married for 22 years)

I feel very sad when I see the normal people who are living better life. Now there is nothing for me, and sometimes I get busy in some work to forget about

> HIV but I can't forget it. When will there be cure; someone has to create the medicine for the cure. Another is I get angry on myself. I don't want to meet the friends. Now there is nothing to live. I want to live normal; I don't want to take medicines. Because of medicine, I feel sleepy also. (Age 36, 12 years of education, never married)

Some men described having no shame or guilt associated with their HIV status:

> No, I do not feel myself guilt and I do not blame on me or others. I am taking my medicine regular and on time, so I follow this timetable regular. I always carry the medicine along with me. Otherwise, I do not think negative or do not have tension of taking medicine. I am very carefree man. (Age 31, nine years of education, married for nine years)

> I didn't felt much bad [after diagnosis], because all my relatives were with me. They were support[ing] me. They know about it, so I didn't get any tension. Now I have my mother, father, 4 children at my home. One daughter got married and one is enough grown to marry. I have lot of support from them. I am earning okay, so there is not much tension in my life. (Age 42, 8 years of education, married for 22 years)

Disclosure

In almost all cases, disclosure was limited to the immediate family. Unmarried men disclosed to parents and siblings; married men primarily to their wives. Men expressed concerns about disclosure that included being blamed for "bad actions," for putting their families at risk and fear that the disease would result in their inability to provide financial support to the household and the loss of *izzat* (respect/honor) in the extended family and community.

> I did not tell [my HIV status] immediately to anybody. But after 6–7 months, I told that to my younger brother. He never approved it. He started scolding me. He said that I must have done something wrong drinking and going to sex workers. He got very angry with me. Then I decided not to tell anybody in the family or others that I am HIV+. If my mother and father come to know about it, they will drive me out of the house. My father is very strict. He will never ever approve or forgive me for having this disease. (Age 24, 14 years of education, married, 1 child)

> Only my wife is aware of my illness. My elder brother and his family stay in in another community. My younger brother also works and stays with them. None

> of them is aware of it. I do not have friends. The workers with whom I work are not that close to discuss such things with them. Nobody else is aware of it. I have not let anybody know about it. (Age 36, 5 years of education, 16 years of marriage, 2 children)

Reaction of Wives

From the in-depth interviews, married men reported that wives had three distinct reactions to the news of their positive HIV status. The first group was supportive, concerned about their husbands and anxious to provide support.

> My wife is very supportive of me; she takes care of me very well. She gives me fresh food, she also asks me every time whether I have taken medicine or not. She also takes care of children very well. Whenever I go to workplace, she insists that I should carry the medicine. Even whenever we go to native place [home village] she carries the medicine from her bag, so that no one can identify that I am taking any such medicine. (Age 34, no education, seven years of marriage, two children)

The more negative responses:

> When I told my wife she also got very angry upon me. She also feels that I must have visited a sex worker. Nobody trusted me. (Age 45, six years of education, two children)

> My wife and my brother-in-law fired on me. My wife told me that you went out for sex and this is the result (*tumne bahar jakar ganda kaam kiya usi ka natija hai ye*). How you get this disease? They blame me a lot that you are not good person. Why you get married if you are having this kind of diseases? You are cheater, you are not good person, and you are *bewda* (drinker) and so many things. I will not excuse you. (Age 37, three years of education, two children)

Several men described that their wives were illiterate and had no knowledge of HIV. This provided them an opportunity to avoid an explanation of the disease and the risks of transmission, using their wives' lack of knowledge to cover the circumstances associated with the acquisition of the disease.

> When doctor told me about my HIV, then I was totally lost. After that doctor told me also to do my wife's testing, but she is illiterate and is unaware of this disease. She agreed to do the test. She is negative and now I have to maintain her status. I don't want her to suffer. Even now, she does not know this disease. (Age 42, 7 years of education, 16 years of marriage, 3 children)

Alcohol and Tensions

Almost all of the men reported that they began consuming alcohol prior to their HIV diagnosis. For some, their AIDS symptoms or the news of diagnosis resulted in a short period of reduction or abstinence only to resume when they became more physically stabilized on ART medication. When asked on the baseline survey why they currently drink, 58.3% chose "to feel happier," 53.0% to have "fun with friends," 45.0% to deal with "tensions," and 30.5% to "forget problems." Alcohol was frequently used to address the tensions associated with their HIV status, their economic situations, family dynamics, and the requirements of the treatment process.

> I tried to reduce drinking alcohol but I could not reduce because sometimes I become tensed and stressed out because of my illness. Then I go and drink *daaru* [alcohol]. Sometimes there is conflict taken place in the family when I come after drinking alcohol. (Age 35, nine years of education, five years of marriage, two children)

> When I feeling tense that time I drink alcohol. I try to ignore the situation when there is tension, stress and guilt feeling, sometimes I cry when I become emotional. Most of the time I try to ignore negative feelings and tension, but if that tension increase then I go alone in the bar and drink alcohol. (Age 33, 10 years of education, never married)

The ART Center

PLHIV are required to pick up their medication on a prearranged day each month incurring transportation costs and the loss of work income from a half to a full day. Medical staff and counselors provide education and examination as PLHIV start on ART, but thereafter the amount of people seeking services precludes more than a cursory review of each PLHIV's medical, educational, and therapeutic needs prior to their receiving their monthly medication. In the in-depth interviews, men complained about a loss of income and transport costs to come to the ART center, the long wait to be processed, and in some cases the negative attitude of the staff.

> They [the ART staff] are not good. They do not do their work fast. Every time we have to stand in the queue for long time. I get irritated to wait in the queue. Every time we have to spend 2–3 hours in the ART center. We have to meet the counselor, doctor and pharmacist to collect medicine. Everywhere we have to stand in the queue. Now I get bored while waiting long for the doctor and collecting medicine thereafter. ART center opens at 9 am, but doctor comes at 10 am. We have to wait for 3–4 hours in the ART center. . . . Sometimes I think I

should stop the medicine because of irritability. (Age 47, 12 years of education, married for 22 years)

Do you think that these staff members [of the ART Center] are working by their choice? Nobody is there to help HIV patients. You should look at their attitude. You should observe the way they interact with the patients. (Age 45, 5 years of education, married for 20 years, 2 children)

While there are complaints, the in-depth interviews document the significance of the ART centers in keeping them healthy:

When I come every month then it is not affordable for me because I have spent more than 40/- rupees. And if I count my working hours, which I spend here then it will go around 200/- rupees. Sometime I feel it is costly but when I think if I take the medicine from private then it will go around more than 5000 rupees which is impossible for me. Also I have to spend for the diet. ART staff told me to eat heavy breakfast, fruits and nutritious foods. (Age 38, 7 years of education, married for 24 years, 1 child)

They [counsellors at ART center] explain my CD4 report; if my CD4 is reduced they ask me to take medicine regular on time. They also ask me to do CD4 test. So the counseling helped me to understand my status of illness, according to that I follow all the precaution. I do not take any tension of my illness, instead of that I am enjoying my life heartily. (Age 51, 9 years of education, married for 26 years)

First thing the counseling which I was provided from the doctor helped me to develop my confidence and it helped me reduce my tension and worries. Then doctor told about food habits so I followed that, I drink milk every day and eat egg, I take my medicine regular and on time, I do not skip a single dose of medicine. I think because of this my CD4 count was increased. (Age 33, 10 years of education, never married)

Alcohol and ART Adherence

The recommendation from ART center counselors and medical staff is that PLHIV should not miss the timing of daily medication. However, it is common that PLHIV in India and elsewhere in the world believe that alcohol and ART medication should not be mixed, either negating the effect of the medication or the mixture causing harm (Kalichman et al. 2009).

If I drink, then my medicine will be of no use. (Age 45, eight years of education, three children, a widow)

I tell others who come to the ART Center that you should not drink before and after taking the medicine. It is very harmful for us. (Age 42, 7, years of education, 16 years of marriage, 3 children)

Doctor told me that taking alcohol and medicines together can damage my liver. (Age 32, 12 years of education, 8 years of marriage, 1 child)

Many men described how they organized their alcohol consumption to not interfere with their medication:

I am very particular about my medicines. I drink only in the evening. After that I I take my medicines and go to sleep. I never go to bed without my medicines. (Age 45, 10 years of education, 25 years of marriage, 5 children)

Usually, I take my medicines at 9:00 am and 9:00 pm. Normally, I drink in the evening at 6:00 pm and finish after one hour. Then after two hours, I take my medicines at my regular time. (Age 44, 15 years of schooling, married for 20 years, 3 children)

The doctor (from the ART Center) says, "Whenever you eat or drink, never fail to take your medicine. That is why I always take my pills with me when I go out and make it a point to purchase a bottle of water and take the medicine on time. Yes I take my pills at the same time as the alcohol. When the alarm rings on my mobile phone, I take the pills from my paper pouch. At that point, my friends [with whom I am drinking] ask what kind of medicine am I taking. I say I am taking medicine for blood pressure." (Age 49, 9 years of education, married for 22 years, 2 children)

Family Concerns

Examples of family concerns included negative relationships with wives, children, and extended family members; household finances; and lack of support for HIV treatment. When the family is at the center of a supportive social environment, concerns about managing HIV treatment and household income are reduced. When the relationship with family is negative and communication is difficult, these concerns weigh heavily on the shoulders of PLHIV.

I don't like having tension and stress. Now I only think that to take care for family, my mother and father, and to educate my son for his good future, to keep my family happy. HIV+ people should not have tension; tension kills the patient!. They should think about their future life and family. (Age 31, nine years of education, married for nine years, one child)

Feelings of guilt and discomfort are exacerbated by social isolation from family members:

> I was in shock because I hadn't thought about this disease and my family members and how they will think about me. Will they accept me or not? It is guilt on my mind and when I stay at home alone then there is some kind of feeling of discomfort. (Age 50, 2 years of education, married for 30 years, 4 children)

External Stigma

Many men described the need to keep their HIV status from their supervisors and coworkers for fear of gossip, taunting, and loss of their job. Some described situations in which the disclosure of their HIV status in the workplace led to job termination.

> The place where I work there is one fellow who is aware about my status; he often visits my *paan*-shop [place for acquiring betel quid with tobacco). Yesterday he came in the evening and he had drunk alcohol, so he was using abusive language using my name. Hence, I was feeling sad, and felt hurt. I used to blame on myself for that. Because of that big mistake, people are behaving with me badly. (Age 35, 10 years of schooling, married, 2 children)

> The Supervisor did not say anything beyond, "Get tested properly. Take your medicines." After that I went to my village. When I returned a few days later, I was fired from my job. (Age 49, six years of schooling, married, two children)

Marriage, Sex, and Children

For single men in their later 20s and early 30s there is great family pressure to marry and have children. For PLHIV who have not disclosed to their extended family, this pressure can be uncomfortable, as relatives keep suggesting candidates for an arranged marriage. In much the same way, families put pressure on married PLHIV men to have children, particularly if the first child is female, creating a dilemma for both concordant and discordant couples. Discordant couples recognize the risk for both wives and children. Concordant couples are concerned about mother-to-child transmission.

> We were clear about our status, and we used contraceptive for safe sex practices, but sometimes I did not use condom, which led to pregnancy and we had our first baby. After first baby, we decided not to have second child by using condom, but even she got pregnant a second time. I do not know, maybe sometimes

I forgot to use condom. Then my mother and father said, the first is girl child, so this time we need boy child. (Age 35, nine years of education, married for five years, two children)

Most of the PLHIV interviewed reported that the diagnosis of HIV, the subsequent complications, and the concern for infecting wives significantly reduced their libido. Hardly any men reported having sex with women who were not their wives. Few single men reported penetrative sex with either women or men. Of 805 men who had wives living with them, 385 (47.8%) reported no sex in the previous year. For 121 married men who reported having sex in the previous month of administration of the baseline survey, 98 (80.2%) used a condom each time they had sex with their wives.

Ever since my diagnosis I never feel urge to have sex [with my wife]. The frequency of our sexual relationship has decreased. Very rarely we indulge in sex. But I am very much cautious that I should not pass on my disease to her, so I use the condom. (Age 48, 10 years of education, married for 22 years, 3 children)

We do not have sex regular but when we have, I use condom every time. If wife is not mentally prepared then I do not force her to have sex. But right now she has lack of interest in sex. I am also not satisfied with [our] sexual life. (Age 34, no education, married for seven years, two children)

I started using condom but every time but she [his wife] was asking why you are using condom now days [she did not understand the disease]. Sometime if I drink more, I also forgot to use condom. (Age 28, seven years of education, married for six years, one child)

I used condoms when I have sex with my wife. Because I have to take care of her, we mostly we do not have sex. I do not want give any kind of tension or disease, which I have in my body. (Age 42, 7 years of education, married for 16 years, 3 children)

My wife is aware about HIV illness, she knows about taking precaution during sexual intercourse. Hence, she does not feel bad about my illness. So we used condom every time during sexual intercourse, and we enjoy and are satisfied with our sex life as like before. (Age 31, 9 years of education, married for 16 years, 3 children)

Sexual intercourse (*jismani rishta*) once in a month is okay for both. Though my religion is against condoms, but I use condom, because I know wife can be infected with HIV if do sex without condom. Mostly both feel satisfied while touching each other [masturbation]. (Age 44, 9 years of education, married for 20 years, 2 children)

DISCUSSION: ART, ALCOHOL, AND HIV AS A CHRONIC ILLNESS

Ekstrand and colleagues (2020), echoing many authors, state, "The global antiretroviral therapy scale-up has been one of the greatest public health success stories in the fight against AIDS, resulting in decreased mortality rates and improved quality of life" (p. 2195). These successes have led advocates to reconceptualize HIV/AIDS as a "chronic disease," as a means to project its manageability, reduce its stigma ("just like heart disease and diabetes"), and to encourage entry into testing and treatment (Calvin 2011; Deeks et al. 2013).

Swendeman and colleagues (2009) characterize chronic disease as prolonged, with a fluctuating course and rarely completely cured. HIV and other chronic diseases in their view share an uncertain course; a prescribed treatment regimen; requirement for self-care; stigma; changes in roles, relationships, and identity; and psychological distress (p. 1322). Heurtin-Roberts and Becker (1993) define chronic diseases as health conditions that can be managed but not cured, with ongoing or periodic symptoms that interfere with daily life.

Does this reconceptualization assist in testing and treatment? Much of the notion of HIV as a chronic disease relates to a relatively narrow biomedical perspective in which ART is able to reduce or achieve an undetectable viral load, reduce the potential for transmission, decrease symptoms and comorbidities, maintain a healthy appearance that reduces interpersonal stigma, and extend the quality and quantity of life. However, ART does not fully restore immunological health and the long-term effects of the disease and the medication can contribute to comorbidities and early aging.

When the focus is beyond the biomedical, it seems clear that HIV comes with significantly more baggage than the typical chronic diseases. From the perspective of the men in this study, the diagnosis of HIV undermines normal life; stigmatizes the individual and the family; requires access to regular and ongoing treatment at less than adequate governmental centers; disrupts marital relationships and sexual life; contributes to the morbidity and mortality of sex partners, wives, and children; affects men's capacity for household support; and contributes to anxiety, tension, stress, and depression. These issues are not easily addressed with one or two daily doses of an ART cocktail.

Anthropologists make a distinction between "disease" and "illness" and "curing" and "healing." Herselman (2007), drawing on this work, defines disease as the "physiological or psychological process of malfunctioning of the body manifest in specific symptoms recognizable by the medical profession, which gives it its identity" (p. 62). In this perspective, the presentation of symptoms, as well as the markers of a low CD4 count and a high viral load, defines seropositive status. Biomedical providers then seek to "cure" or at least mitigate the disease by focusing on the treatment (alteration) of the pathological processes that cause the symptoms. This disease-curative approach defines most of the treatment process for PLHIV in ART centers in greater Mumbai and elsewhere.

However, what about the structural, social, and psychological issues that continue to disrupt the lives of most of the men in this chapter? These issues require the need to address the illness-healing (emic) components of the anthropological construct. "Illness" can be defined as the individuals' "subjective experiences and interpretations of sickness in line with their health belief system rooted in their culture (Herselman 2007, p. 62)." From another perspective, sickness is not only in the individual but disrupts the equilibrium of the family, the social network, the community, and the society. To address these illness issues requires "healing," that is, going beyond biomedical intervention and the curative process to address the psychological, social, and societal impacts of the illness.

For the men in this study, alcohol raises an additional illness component and a complication of both curing and healing. The literature over the past decade has consistently identified the negative effects of alcohol on immune status, comorbidities, transmission risk, medication adherence, and psychological status. For the most part, ART centers in LMICs and in India do not regularly address alcohol consumption. Alcohol use brings with it its own stigma in the cultural context of India where there are negative attitudes toward public consumption and inebriation and a perceived link to men who seek commercial sex. In the family context, alcohol consumption by PLHIV affects the role of men as financial supporter of the household, continuing the behaviors that led to HIV infection, disrupting spousal and familial relationships, undermining ART medication, providing a dysfunctional approach to internalized guilt and stigma, and limiting the ability to cope with complex relationships within family and society.

ART is a necessary but not sufficient element of a comprehensive healing approach. What is needed is the recognition that PLHIV must own the healing process if the illness is to be fully addressed. Because of limited resources and overcrowding, much of current HIV treatment in ART centers in India and other LMICs is limited to medication pickup. A comprehensive healing approach requires addressing the issues and challenges that contribute to the physical and emotional health of PLHIV and in particular, to those who consume alcohol. A first component of that comprehensive approach involves expanding knowledge concerning healthy living, ART medication, the negative impact of alcohol, the importance of social and familial support, and the resources available to address new and ongoing issues. A second component involves the need to address internalized stigma that includes the guilt and shame of disease etiology that can lead to dysfunctional actions, including lack of disclosure to people who can help, isolation, and alcohol consumption. A third component involves the creation of relationships with other PLHIV to share common problems and potential solutions. A fourth component is participation in efforts to address the structural issues of societal stigma, ensure PLHIV entitlements established by the GOI, and address discriminatory practices of public and private institutions by PLHIV.

The NIAAA/NIH project utilized the in-depth interviews, the baseline survey, and the observation of the functioning of the ART programs to design a comprehensive, multilevel and multidimensional approach to the healing process. Interventions consisted of individual counseling, group intervention, and collective advocacy focused on healthy living, tension and anxiety, alcohol, ART adherence, and relationships. Collective advocacy was based on the premise that participation in structural change would increase the sense of empowerment of PLHIV to manage HIV and the associated work, family, and psychological issues. The results showed that the interventions, singly and in sequence, had a significant impact on the key healing indicators (Singh et al. 2020).

HIV/AIDS programs conducted in India are barely keeping up with the provision and distribution of ART medication and sustaining additional services seems not realistic. A coalition of positive peoples' groups, other governmental entities and NGOs, and PLHIV can deliver multiple healing components. All illnesses require a healing rather than just a curative process; HIV/AIDS, both globally and in India, needs a more comprehensive approach to address the needs of PLHIV. The terminology of "chronicity" and the expectation of the "end" to AIDS will provide little help; a healing coalition working with and beyond ART centers can produce the action necessary to address the healing process.

NOTE

1. I am grateful to my fellow principal investigators, Drs. Niranjan Saggurti and Avina Sarna of India Country Office of the Population Council, Ravi Verma of the Asia Regional Office of the International Center for Research on Women (ICRW), and Jean J. Schensul of Institute for Community Research, Hartford, Connecticut, for their

collaboration on this project. The day-to-day operations of data collection and intervention rested on the skills and management of the project coordinators, Dr. Melita Vaz of Population Council, Dr. Priti Prabhughate, Rajendra Singh, and Parasnath Verma of ICRW, and our tireless staff of research investigators and interventionists. This study depended on the support of National AIDS Control Organization, the Maharashtra State AIDS Control Society, the Mumbai District AIDS Control Society, the leaders of the five participating hospitals, and the staff of the ART centers. Lastly, I would like to thank study participants who willingly gave us their time and attention.

REFERENCES

Colvin, CJ 2011. HIV/AIDS, chronic disease and globalization. *Globalization and Health* 7, no. 31: 1–6.

Chawla R, Ichhpujani RL 2011. Enteric spore-forming opportunistic parasites in HIV/AIDS. *Tropical Parasitology*, 1, no. 1, 15–19.

Deeks S, Lewin S and Havlir D 2013. The End of AIDS: HIV Infection as a chronic disease. *Lancet* 382, no. 9903, 1525–1533.

Ekstrand ML, Heylen E, Periera M, D'Souza J, Nair S, Mazur A, Shamsundar R, Kumar BNR, Chandy S 2020. A behavioral adherence intervention improves rates of viral suppression among adherence challenged people living with HIV in South India. *AIDS and Behaviour* 24, no. 7, 2195–2205.

Fauci AS, Folkers GK. 2012. Toward an AIDS-free generation. *JAMA* 308, no. 4, 1529–36.

Ha T, Schensul SL, Irving M, Brault MA, Schensul JJ, Prabhughate P, Vaz M. 2018. Depression among Alcohol Consuming, HIV Positive Men on ART Treatment in India. *AIDS Behaviour* 23, no. 6, 1623–1633.

Herselman S. 2007. Health care through a cultural lens: Insights from medical anthropology. *Current allergy and Clinical Immunology* 20, no. 1, 62–65.

Heurtin-Roberts S and Becker G. 1993. Anthropological Perspectives on Chronic illness. *Social Science and Medicine* 37, 281–283.

Kalichman SC, Grebler T, Amaral CM, McNerey M, White D, Kalichman MO, Cherry C, Eaton L. 2013. Intentional non-adherence to medications among HIV positive alcohol drinkers: prospective study of interactive toxicity beliefs. *Journal of General Internal Medicine*, 28 no. 3, 399–405.

Kalichman S, Amaral CM, White D, Swetsze C, Pope H, Kalichman MO, Cherry C, and Eaton L. 2009. Prevalence and clinical implications of interactive toxicity beliefs regarding mixing alcohol and antiretroviral therapies among people with HIV/AIDS. *AIDS Patient Care and STDs* 23, no. 6, 449–454.

Levi J, Raymond A, Pozniak A, et al. 2016. Can the UNAIDS 90-90-90 target be achieved? A systematic analysis of national HIV treatment cascades. *BMJ Global Health* 1, no. 2, 1–10.

Sangaramoorthy T. 2018. Chronicity, crisis, and the 'end of AIDS.' *Global Public Health* 13, no. 8, 982–996.

National AIDS Control Organization: Facts and Figures 2017. Accessed on September 12, 2020. http://naco.gov.in/hiv-facts-figures

Pizzoli SFM, Renzi C, Arnaboldi P, Russel-Edu W, Pravetti G. 2019. From life threatening to chronic disease; Is this the case of cancers? A systematic review. *Cogent Psychology* 6, no.1, 1–17.

Schensul SL, Ha T, Schensul JJ, Vaz M, Singh R, Burleson JA, Bryant K. 2017.The Role of Alcohol on Antiretroviral Therapy Adherence among Persons Living With HIV in Urban India. *Journal of Studies on Alcohol and Drugs* 78, no. 5, 716–724.

Singh RJ, Sarna A, Schensul JJ, Mahapatra B, Ha T, Schensul SL. 2020. A multilevel intervention to reduce stigma among alcohol consuming men living with HIV receiving antiretroviral therapy: findings from a randomized control trial in India. *AIDS* 1, no. 34 Suppl. 1, S83–S92.

Stringer, KL, Marotta P, Baker E, Turan, B, Kempf MC, Drentea P, Turan JM., 2019. Substance Use Stigma and Antiretroviral Therapy Adherence Among a Drug-Using Population Living with HIV. *AIDS Patient Care STDS* 33, no. 6, 282–293.

Swendam D, Ingram B, and Rotheram-Borus, MJ. 2009. Common elements in self-management of HIV and other chronic diseases: an integrative framework. *AIDS Care* 21, no. 10, 1321–1334.

UNAIDS 2014. 90-90-90: An ambitious treatment target to help end the AIDS epidemic. Accessed on September 10, 2020. https://www.unaids.org/sites/default/files/media_asset/90-90-90_en.pdf

Williams, EC, McGinnis KA, Edelman, EJ, Matson TE, Gordon AJ, Marshall BD, Bradley KA. 2019. Level of Alcohol Use Associated with HIV Care Continuum Targets in a National U.S. Sample of Persons Living with HIV Receiving Healthcare. *AIDS Behaviour* 23, no. 1, 140–151.

Yadav D, Chakrapani V, Goswami P, Ramanathan S, Ramakrishnan L, George B, Paranjape RS. 2014. Association between alcohol use and HIV-related sexual risk behaviors among men who have sex with men (MSM): findings from a multi-site bio-behavioral survey in India. *AIDS Behaviour* 18, no. 7, 1330–1338.

Conclusion

Remembering HIV in the Era of Eradication: Critical Nostalgia, Infrastructures of Accountability, and the Fate of Viral Socialities

Robert Lorway

The chapters in this collection appear at a time of "HIV optimism" expressed over the possibility of an "AIDS-free future" (Sangaranoorthy 2018, Kenworthy et al. 2018). Yet the authors' stories paint quite a different picture, playing to a sense of tragic irony: delegitimated guardians in Uganda (Walsh Lang), morally rejected experimental subjects in Egypt (Hassan), pathologizing public health discourses in Caribbean (Jolly), and excluded access to safe, nondiscriminatory care in India, South Africa, and Canada (Saria, Ordóñez, Schensul, and Murray). At face, these haunting stories present all-too-familiar and enduring tales of stigmatization in the history of HIV. Moreover, they seem to raise the rather pointed question: HIV optimism—for whom and in whose interest? What transformations can people living with HIV actually claim in the era of biomedical advancement, especially those living under the weight of structural violence and poverty, statist forms of nationalist oppression, and moralistic normativities wrought by public health interventions? How do we make sense of this moment, if indeed it is somehow "transformed"?

Attempting to examine this larger question in relation to the chapters has thrown my sense of ethnographic recollection "out of time" in ways that join with Murray's discussion of nostalgia and temporality. I began thinking back to my own work in the early 1990s with the AIDS Coalition of Nova Scotia in eastern Canada, as a local researcher, community health volunteer, acting sexually transmitted infections clinical manager, and outreach worker—in the years before highly active antiretrovirals were discovered in North America, when young gay men were coming home to die from large urban centers to smaller towns. For the first time, many of these men were coming out to their families about their sexual alterity, about being infected with a stigmatizing virus, and about facing what was then only known as a terminal illness. In the 1980s and early 1990s, science had very few answers in terms of treatment; the initial overprescription of AZT as a highly ineffective monotherapy, which actually hastened some deaths, only further sowed the seeds of doubt in biomedicine and science. Discrimination against people living with HIV and dying of AIDS in hospitals fostered deep distrust in the health care system. The memory returns to me of nursing staff abruptly dropping food trays while hurriedly exiting the isolated hospital rooms in palliative care. Many of these same health professionals also marked those of us volunteering in these isolated spaces with the same brush of untouchability. I still hear the words of nurses discussing our group of volunteers who were assisting with patient feedings, one of them referring to us as "*Those* AIDS people," clearly knowing that we were within earshot. HIV stigma was highly reactive then, igniting its own "epidemic of signification," to borrow words from cultural studies scholar Paula Treichler (1999), while fueling a wider field of inflamed politics surrounding homophobia, racism, whorephobia, and xenophobia. Provincial political leaders in my home province, who were years too late in their response to the epidemic, were also highly reluctant to touch an epidemic that was seemingly confined to the most reviled in society.

I am also reminded, however, that as tragic as these times were in terms of myriad struggles that people endured in their families, workplaces, and the health care system—this period saw the vibrant emergence of highly nourishing forms of sociality that unfurled around HIV as a social justice project. Importantly, the existence of pronounced scientific uncertainty and health systems failure that marked HIV-related oppressions provided fertile terrain for this thriving biosociality to grow. As Stephen Epstein (1996) compellingly chronicles, powerful forms of lay expertise rose to confront scientists on their own territories in the absence of a cure, lack of effective treatment, and widespread systemic discrimination in health care systems. Grassroots authority over community health powerfully mobilized as health activists set up innovative systems of health service delivery, hospice care, and education and prevention programs, which worked along the same channels as their intimate social connections with each other, while at the same time reshaping the edges of health and social service institutions. Grassroots resources, steeped in liberal feminist, queer, antiracist ideologies, served the benefit not only of communities of people living with HIV neglected by the health care system, but these resources were also placed at the disposal of the wider public, which was paramount to the response when women's HIV prevalence in Canada dramatically rose in the early 1990s. Governments and health officials eventually began to invest in grassroots health initiatives with the growing recognition that community action and health promotion effectively tempered the ills that stigma presented to health care access and well-being.

It seems important to remember that this period of scientific uncertainty, doubt, mistrust, failure, and even pessimism produced dynamic and politically inflected forms of care that gave HIV its "lively" quality: a microscopic virus, and the inability of science to halt its transmission, drew many of us together into highly affected and widely reaching communities, whether HIV infected or not. Struggles to confront ongoing discrimination and moral panic during this period not only quickly incited widespread forms of grassroots politicization, but the very practices of politicization—that is, thinking and doing politically—which had so much room to flourish amid uncertainty and failure, formed the very connective strands in ways of caring for each other. For people confronting HIV and AIDS, this enabled them to live well on their own terms. The possibility and flourishment of these kinds of "viral socialities" are what seem, to me, to be at stake in this "End of AIDS" era of optimism. Borrowing the notion of "viral socialities" from Fadhila Mazanderani's (2012) discussion of the "broader ethics of intimacy" within the context of sexual relationships, I invoke this notion here more with respect to the affective, intimate ties that form between groups of people as they confront the lived effects of denigration, deprivation, and injustices attaching to the array of sociopolitical meanings that imbued HIV as a stigmatizing illness.

Although it may be tempting to read the various forms of stigma portrayed in the preceding chapters as the persistence of a long, continuous, and familiar global story in the history of AIDS, it is important to recognize that there are many critical ruptures at play in our current era, plagued by what I would call *the will to intervene*. This notion resembles João Biehl's (2009) *Will to Live* insomuch as it gestures toward particular biopolitical impulses that maintain the life processes of "the population" at the center of political discourse. However, rather than seeing a shift away from "prevention" toward "equal access," which has, in the case of Brazil, reconfigured an "activist state" out of particular alliances between HIV activists, health professionals, and state and private sector actors (Biehl 2009), we are witnessing the intensification of techno-bureaucratic power arrangements that (1) move to diminish the unruly force of activist visions of the future, which are caught up in affective dispositions toward struggle and crisis and (2) intensify anticipatory prevention logics (Adams, Murphy, and Clarke 2009). As a later form of neoliberal state governance, the will to intervene recasts the future as something that can be efficiently and sedately managed, calculated, measured, and achieved through adherence to procedures, guidelines, milestones, and targets. This course invests in the agency of technicians (epidemiologic, monitoring and evaluation specialists, program designers and managers, mathematical modelers and forecasters, policy makers, health professionals, and health officials) over and above activists in the imaginary of HIV eradication. Yet, the returns on the investment in the will to intervene have unleashed their own highly charged affective biopolitical terrain.

As many of the chapters show, we are now confronted with new forms of technocratic violence that move to "obscure an on-going crisis" (Sangaramoorthy 2018)—a form of violence wrought by the intensified momentum of transnational efforts to create "AIDS free futures." Therefore, my localized starting point in briefly recollecting HIV's history of uncertainty, failure, and neglect—while pointing toward the notion of viral socialities—is intended as a form of "critical nostalgia" (Cashman 2006) to underscore and reimagine different possibilities in a present that appears hyper-focused on technocratic response, in a reactive way that diminishes attention to the broader role of structural violence and inequality. Critical questions remain with respect to the moment of optimism we have entered, a moment which overemphasizes eradication as the central unproblematic goal of health futurity and wellness in relation to HIV.

Amid declarations of scientific "success" in terms of clinical efficacy and "real-world" demonstrations of effectiveness around HAART; prevention of vertical (mother-to-child) transmission of HIV; treatment as prevention (decreasing viral load to undetectable levels to reduce transmission in a given population); and, most notably, PrEP (and CAB LA,[1] and various other long-acting injectables on the eve of their release), many health scientists today would claim we have entered an era of certainty. Taken together, these scientific advances present, it would seem, a defining moment of profound redemption for science—a long-awaited relief from its previous history of failure and uncertainty. Giving rise to an optimism and an imaginary of an "AIDS free future," the notion of "eradication" resounds in global health policy in recent years. For what could stand in the way of the seemingly straightforward biomedical solution of getting these efficacious, portable, and increasingly available substances into bodies?

While many of the chapters in this collection join a larger chorus in critical studies of health and development that reiterate how the delivery of highly efficacious health technologies rarely follows a straightforward path, they also edge us toward acknowledging the excitability of the very notion of eradication itself. Appearing closer on the horizon, as though within reach, the futurity of "end of AIDS" has ushered in an aggressive pragmatism in the present that leaves little time for responders to contemplate the crucial role that localized "viral socialities" might play in supporting much broader visions of what it means to live well (and not just with HIV).[2] Here I am talking about the global health apparatus that makes its appearance, in one way or another, in many of the chapters. To more fully understand how people living with HIV experience stigma, I insist, we must pay close attention, as some of the authors do, to what I would call the "infrastructures of accountability" that appropriate more and more territory under the public health gaze. HIV stigma, in other words, not only grows out of forms of negation (e.g., of marginalization, exclusion, and neglect), but it is also powerfully and productively instantiated in and through "the will to intervene" and the rapidly expanding infrastructures of accountability established to "end AIDS."

In recent discussions with community activists, peer outreach workers, and their allied health scientists and health officials in India and Kenya, I have learned how the global strategy of "treatment as prevention," 90-90-90 (now accelerated to "95-95-95") and U=U, has unleashed new moral panics over what I am now repeatedly hearing: "Find the positives!"—a mantra that joins with pledge made in the Sustainable Development Goals to "leave no one behind" (UNDP 2020). This new public health imperative of targeting and finding HIV+ people stirs up existential questions for community-led organizations whose funding futures and political survival depend upon reaching these newly prescribed targets set by Western-oriented multilateral donors such as the Global Fund, USAID, CDC, and PEPFAR. In other words, we have seen a profound linguistic and affective shift from directing responders to connect with people to reduce stigma (to safely connect them to vital health services) via community health promotion actors and narratives to "finding the positives," as though HIV were an entity isolatable from the dense solidarities of viral socialities that nourish the health and well-being of people. In other words, eradication narratives, furnished by the global health apparatus, unleash a biopolitical regime that reduces bodies to targets of pathogenic containment, while simultaneously opening up biosocial intimacies to the aggressive disciplining impulses of population health logics of funding allocation, accountability, and expediency.

As many of these chapters show, in the name of realizing an "AIDS-free future" and "health improvement," we are witnessing the expansion of ever more extensive projects of intervention and surveillance that go well beyond the clinic proper. This is vividly portrayed in Walsh Lang's study of ARV treatment adherence programs in South Africa for children with HIV and AIDS: the most intimate spheres of kinship and family are interpellated into a technocratic regime that governs children's access to health services, nutrition, education, and even place of residence. These broad spheres of living are regulated through the routine tracking of a series of narrowly construed indicators that measure biological and behavioral markers. These highly decontextualizing indicators—and the unquestioned graduated normativities they impart—allow to flourish a technocratic rendition of care "by numbers" (Shore and Wright 2015) in ways that circumvent any fuller reckoning with structural rootings and social exclusions people are unable to escape. As Walsh Lang's chapter suggests, this enumerative regime resigns people, both children and their "unworthy" parents, to live out conflicted and even tormented lived realities in silence and out of public sight. To me, this exemplifies the new conditions of HIV stigma in the "eradication era": What does it mean to live with HIV, and to live "positively" in the shadows created by success? Does one's very embodied existence as an HIV+ person increasingly take on the material semiotic presence of failure? Are people living with HIV becoming "the abject" (Kristeva 1982), left to haunt the outer edges of precision-oriented modern technocratic systems of HIV "innovation" such that it becomes possible (and somehow "reasonable") in instances of long-term survival to ask the disturbing question posed by the doctor in Toronto to Murray's interlocutors: "Aren't you people all dead?"

Violent stigmatization that forms in the shadows created by the drive to realize success and the impetus to intervene is also illuminated by Hassan with respect to Egypt. In this case, celebrations of a device that supposedly can cure people bring HIV optimism into an unexpected and deeply unsettling alliance with a militarized nationalism. The effort to publicly restage "the cure" in Egypt places the physical bodies of people living with HIV at the center of this biopolitical configuration, and does so by licensing highly invasive biomedical experiments on people living with HIV that produce dire outcomes. At the same time, the moral contest orchestrated by the military experimental protocols, which separates "the innocent" people living with HIV from "the guilty," sacrifices the possibility of greater unity between people living with HIV. These discriminations enacted by state actors erode, even before they may form, the very possibility of flourishing viral socialities that could help ease the morally fraught experience of living with HIV in Egypt—further reestablishing political power over citizens in a postrevolutionary (2011–2014) demonstration of nationalism. Social stigma, moral condemnation by the state, and profound isolation and distrust do not stand apart from or flee this vehement biopolitical project of staging conquest over HIV. Rather, stigma is instrumentalized to erect what Saria aptly refers to in their chapter as "fantasies of the state," and thereby remakes the boundaries of moral citizenship in hetero-masculinist terms.

With actually few options for accessing lifesaving and affirming programs, participation of poorer Egyptians in these physically extensive and highly risky experiments becomes a reasonable option for them as disenfranchised people. Resorting to participation in experiments to access a greater level of care and quality of health services (also see Petryna 2007, Nguyen 2009), in Hassan's case, in some ways parallels how the vulnerabilities of people with HIV in West African locations are harnessed for Ebola vaccine trial objectives. As Thiongane and Graham's chapter shows, clinical trial practices bend the logic of CD4 cell count measurements in order to justify the testing and retesting of potential subjects until they can fit within the inclusion criteria.

Without access to quality health care, many of these participants are effectively manipulated into achieving the goals of the trial scientists that take precedence over the goal of safety—what the CD4 guidelines were originally intended to ensure.

In these examples, it is important to take note, with respect to routine program monitoring and experimental protocols, how the materiality of HIV+ bodies in "end of AIDS" projects accrues surplus value or "biovalue" (Waldby 2002; Rajan 2006) in regimes of tracking, measuring, and engaging those who have come to be known in public health policy parlance as "key" or "priority" populations. And as streams of global health funding come to increasingly rely upon the continuous measurements of HIV+ bodies, people living with HIV become ever more entangled in economies of accountability. A number of the chapters call out the ways in which these regimes unfairly off-load responsibility onto "the individual," often blaming people living with HIV for the persistence of new infections and the failure of prevention and treatment programs. This criticism is tied to the decontextualizing effects of the public health apparatus. Here, however, I want to suggest that as ethnographers we may need to push further in our critical examination of this technical apparatus and epistemic formation by treating public health infrastructures of accountability as a complex lead character, one that performs double duty in tracking and reporting new infections and program outcomes while also enabling funders to track the returns on their investments (Erikson 2012, 2019; Lorway and Khan 2014). I would argue that these infrastructures erase contextual realities that may be important to understand what might be missing from contemporary practices of care in the field of HIV. But in teasing apart the complex workings of these infrastructures of accountability and the logics they disseminate, we may begin to better understand how countries elaborately and effectively are made accountable, in a broader sense, to the transnational project of "getting to zero," as enshrined in the 2011 UNAIDS initiative and other normative global health development policies.

Global health reporting systems that track people's linkage to testing, treatment, and adherence along the prevention-treatment continuum of care, especially those that converge in low- and middle-income countries, operate according to their own temporal rhythms that may be out of step with the pace of lived realities of people accessing services (Benton et al. 2017). I would add to this point that these reporting systems greatly affect those working in technical capacities along service delivering pathways (and by "reporting systems" here I am specifically referring to the interlocking health administration-informational systems that collate clinical, epidemiological, and program data and other information from highly systemized monitoring, evaluation, and outreach schemes that target "key populations"). Elsewhere

I've written about how an array of technical experts deploy standardizing enumerative technologies like geographic mapping, microplanning, form filling, and so on, giving rise to exchanges of population size estimates and denominators between governmental HIV units and multilateral funding agencies—creating a global political economy of metrics that circumscribes certain conditions of possibility for civil society entities such as community-based organizations, many of which historically have been the major custodians of care for people living with HIV (Lorway 2021). Thinking about the animation of this system of reporting along the lines that Adia Benton, Thurka Sangaramoorthy, and Ippolytos Kalofonos (2017) have with respect to what they refer to as "project time," I am led to also wonder about how "reporting time" mobilizes temporal orientations of futurity in the present and affective dispositions of hope and failure among those embedded in various locations within these terrains of health administration, monitoring, and evaluation. How do these diverse knowledge workers' anxieties play into and out from nationalist insecurities, thereby driving the pace of their efforts to meet the daunting task of generating the country's portrait of an HIV epidemic, one which determines a country's ranking on a global scale of progress?

The powerful and complicated role that public health infrastructures play in delaying and interrupting "universal" ARV access among India's poor living with HIV, as vividly depicted by Saria, cautions us to realize the susceptibility of infrastructures to wider political maneuvers of the state (like Hassan), which, as Saria shows, manufactures the crisis of ARV shortages, despite India's reputedly flexible and conducive regulatory climate surrounding generic drug production, so as to continue to capture streams of global health funding. Furthermore, the supply chain management system takes on the all-too-familiar appearance of inefficient bureaucratic forms that plague the administration of health and social services to India's poor and unleash widespread structural violence (Gupta 2012). Physicians working in this system of frequent delays and shortages are forced to continually improvise the clinical care they provide, twisting accepted protocols beyond recognition, it would seem. At the same time, responsibility for nonadherence often gets displaced onto the poor, without any fuller acknowledgment of how the very conditions of poverty contribute to nonadherence. What are the possibilities for living positively within a public health system that is not only mired in bureaucratic efficiencies but which also, simultaneously, holds impoverished patients accountable for their own failures? Moreover, the persistence of a clearly broken public health system in India, perhaps by design, is premised on the more general illusion of poor people living with HIV while enjoying forms of wellness—a recurring mirage of "ARV access" and positive living, which vanishes as quickly as it appears for them.

The problems of infrastructural expansion in the age of biomedical advancement not only invisibilize the exigencies of daily life for impoverished people living with HIV in low- or middle-income countries, but also in economically more privileged settings like Toronto, Canada, as Murray's chapter illuminates, people living with HIV are left to contend with health services delivery modalities that have become "increasingly bureaucratized through gradual enmeshment in the state funded public health system" (page 157). As Murray's interlocutors recount, programs running at HASOs only serve to distance them from their own deeply rooted and temporally inflected lived histories of HIV and social change. For this group of aging, long-term "survivors" who lived through the triumphs of activism that birthed new forms of community health promotion and permitted viral socialities to extend into the very recesses of service delivery and "community-friendly" clinical practice, they are now forced to grapple with forms of spatial dispossession as they enter the very places they were once instrumental in creating for the benefit of all people living with HIV in Canada. It appears that this new version of "progress" in the era of prevention's success and "population level disease control" leaves little room for these protective and health affirming social textures to thrive. Moreover, the very presence of these long-term survivors appears to disrupt the performativity of progress that gained its momentum along the road to scientific redemption. In a new system that is fully embraced by biomedicine and the pharmaceuticalization of HIV care for gay men, these older figures of activist life and viral sociality lose their recognition and value; they inhabit the fringes—invisibilized to an archives that science seems determined to forget. But this state of invisibility and marginalization is not a mere return to a prior state of stigma or the continuation of the crisis, as some scholars might contend. Oppressions endured by people living with HIV today are produced in a profoundly transformed way. Violence is enacted not only through blatant discrimination and denial but much more insidiously through the quiet, silent dissemination of pages for form filling, bureaucratic processing, and standardize templates making, that is, practices that reduce complex experiences to simplified data points. It is important to underscore Murray's point concerning the neglect shown by HASOs toward people living with HIV, as it reveals the shadowy underside of the biopolitical will to intervene and "to make live" (Lemke 2011)—long-term survivors become those who can be let go of, as though undeserving of care.

This bureaucratic violence—in its mundaneness, repetition, rigidity, and silence—is indeed a much harder political object to confront and politicize than forms of outright discrimination, which helps to explain the kind of melancholic nostalgia expressed by Murray's interlocutors whose dissent seemed confined to private meetings of their support group. At the same time, I am also left to wonder—are these discussions of disillusionment perhaps also the scattered seeds of pre- or new political or activist formations in unrealized futures, yet to come? When read alongside Jolly's chapter, the political possibilities of resilient, intimate, and persistent viral socialities in the face of global health regimes and infrastructures of accountability become especially apparent. Jolly shows how communities of Black women living with HIV in Jamaica, although greatly overlooked as important political actors in the history of HIV activism, have created their own intimate communities of care and support, living out daily realities that release bodies from the biomedical confinements presumed of illness. Mobilizing, instead, "the erotic," as Audre Lorde does in her writings, Jolly shows how "counter modes of intimacy and self-presentation offer possibilities for marginalized women to carve out space for self-making beyond the delimited sites of public health and HIV advocacy" (page 174)—defying them in ways that remake the disciplining logics of individual responsibility and morality into transcendent and nourishing collective-care-making lived realities. Although traceable to Caribbean women's longer histories of weaving together forms of political change through the ordinary and available fabrics of quotidian life, as Jolly reminds us, there are important reminders here of the continued crucial relevance of forms of HIV activism that politicize sexuality, desire, and pleasure even at a time of ubiquitous techno-bureaucratic articulations of global health governance.

Looking across the papers, despite the looming presence of HIV eradication narratives, indeed we see various forms of intimacy and flourishment, that stubbornly persist and endure. The very act of these anthropologists to dwell on what it means to live with HIV in ways that disrupt global health scientific normativities and biomedical claims of certainty are themselves highly promising political interventions. What critical possibilities exist in looking back, forward, and across temporalities and geographies, as we've been able to do in these chapters, and what might these perspectives hold for emergent forms of political and activist remakings?

NOTES

1. A long-acting injectable prophylaxis.
2. Here my thinking borrows from Peter Redfield's (2013) ethnographic study of Médecins sans Frontieres and his notion of how humanitarian declarations of urgency and crisis are driven by an "emphasis on action over contemplation" (p. 3).

REFERENCES

Adams, Vincanne, Michelle Murphy, and Adele E. Clarke. 2009. "Anticipation: Technoscience, Life, Affect, Temporality." *Subjectivity* 28 (1): 246–265.

Benton, Adia, Thurka Sangaramoorthy, and Ippolytos Kalofonos. 2017. "Temporality and Positive Living in the Age of HIV/AIDS—A Multi-Sited Ethnography." *Current Anthropology* 58 (4): 454–476.

Biehl, João. 2009. *Will to Live: AIDS Therapies and the Politics of Survival.* Princeton, NJ: Princeton University Press.

Cashman, Ray. 2006. "Critical Nostalgia and Material Culture in Northern Ireland." *Journal of American Folklore* 119 (472): 137–160.

Epstein, Stephen. 1996. *Impure Science: AIDS, Activism, and the Politics of Knowledge*. Berkeley: University of California Press.

Erikson, Susan L. 2012. "Global Health Business: The Production and Performativity of Statistics in Sierra Leone and Germany." *Medical Anthropology* 31 (4): 367–384.

Erikson, Susan. 2019. "Global Health Futures?: Reckoning with a Pandemic Bond." *Medicine Anthropology Theory* 6 (3): 77–108.

Gupta, Akhil. 2012. *Red Tape: Bureaucracy, Structural Violence, and Poverty in India*. Durham: Duke University Press.

Kenworthy, Nora, Matthew Thomann, and Richard Parker. 2018. "From a Global Crisis to the 'End of AIDS': New Epidemics of Signification." *Global Public Health* 13 (8): 960–971.

Kristeva, Julia. 1982. "Approaching Abjection." *Oxford Literary Review* 5 (1\2): 125–149.

Lemke, Thomas. 2011. "Beyond Foucault." In *Governmentality. Current Issues and Future Challenges*, edited by Ulrich Bröckling, Susanne Krasmann, Thomas Lemke, 65–184. New York: Routledge.

Lorway, Robert. 2021. "Check Your Denominator: Geographic Mapping, Activism and the Standardization of Sexual Risk." In *The Social Life of Standards,* edited by Janice Graham, Christina Holmes, Fiona McDonald, and Regna Darnell, 114–137. Vancouver: University of British Columbia Press.

Lorway, Robert, and Shamshad Khan. 2014. "Reassembling Epidemiology: Mapping, Monitoring and Making-up People in the Context of HIV Prevention in India." *Social Science & Medicine* 112: 51–62.

Mazanderani, Fadhila. 2012. "An Ethics of Intimacy: Online Dating, Viral-Sociality and Living with HIV." *BioSocieties* 7 (4): 393–409.

Nguyen, Vinh-Kim. 2009. "Government-by-Exception: Enrolment and Experimentality in Mass HIV Treatment Programmes in Africa." *Social Theory & Health* 7 (3): 196–217.

Petryna, Adriana. 2007. "Experimentality: On the Global Mobility and Regulation of Human Subjects Research." *PoLAR: Political and Legal Anthropology Review* 30 (2): 288–304.

Rajan, Kaushik Sunder. 2006. *Biocapital: The Constitution of Postgenomic Life*. Durham: Duke University Press.

Redfield, Peter. 2013. *Life in Crisis: The Ethical Journey of Doctors Without Borders*. Berkeley: University of California Press.

Sangaramoorthy, Thurka. 2018. "Chronicity, Crisis, and the 'End of AIDS'." *Global Public Health* 13 (8): 982–996.

Shore, Cris and Wright, Susan. 2015. "Governing by Numbers: Audit Culture, Rankings and the New World Order." *Social Anthropology* 23 (1): 22–28.

Treichler, Paula A. 1999. *How to Have Theory in an Epidemic: Cultural Chronicles of AIDS*. Durham: Duke University Press.

UNDP. 2020. "Leaving No One Behind." https://sustainabledevelopment.un.org/content/documents/2754713_July_PM_2._Leaving_no_one_behind_Summary_from_UN_Committee_for_Development_Policy.pdf

Waldby, Catherine. 2002. "Stem Cells, Tissue Cultures and the Production of Biovalue." *Health* 6 (3): 305–323.

Afterword

Beyond the Endgame?

Adia Benton

In 2015, UNAIDS announced an ambitious agenda: to end AIDS as a public health threat by 2030 (heretofore glossed as "the end of AIDS"). A series of mathematical models have intimated that "the end of AIDS" can be achieved via a 90-90-90 approach, that is: if 90% of the (estimated) 37 million people in the world living with HIV learn their HIV serostatus, if 90% of them initiate antiretroviral therapies, and if 90% of treated people maintain an undetectable load, beginning in 2020, we could see the end of HIV/AIDS as a public health problem in a 10-year period. Ten years!

That's a lot of ifs.

Given that those "ifs" appear to be based upon big fractions with shifty denominators, the labor required to transform them into reality (the "is") across a wide range of political, social, and economic contexts and levels will be herculean. Managerial expressions like "90-90-90" and "end of AIDS by 2030" are policy thresholds deemed achievable, realistic, and measurable within a specified timeframe. Such thresholds are the bread and butter of international governance. They standardize and normalize appropriate processes and actions for change in the realm of HIV/AIDS, allowing for commensuration and synchronization of HIV programming—shared common ground and, hopefully, commensurate resources—across national, regional, and global scales. These metrics give HIV workers something to aspire to, something tangible to intervene upon, if not fail toward.

But as most technocrats and others involved in managing and mitigating the impact of our AIDS pandemic know, the process for reaching the numerical benchmarks indexed by "90-90-90," the everyday experience of HIV/AIDS and its management across abstract sites (like communities, localities, nation-states) and real bodies, in particular places and times, is where "if" and "is" are in constant tension. *If* the vast majority are tested, *if* the vast majority are treated, *if* their viral loads remain suppressed, the gap between "if" and "is" widens along the fault lines of inequality and manifold oppressions.

As the gap between "if" and "is" narrows, as they inch toward each other—and I believe this is implied in the very goal of ending AIDS—the tension between "if" and "is" of HIV/AIDS prevention, treatment, and care will continue to be productive. They have already produced what I, following myriad others, have described as HIV exceptionalism: disease-specific bureaucratic and administrative relationships that reconfigured social, political, and economic relations in service of lofty goals and HIV's exceptional status. They have also reproduced many of the inequalities that set HIV's exceptionalism in motion. This has implications for whether those ifs can be—or should be—the basis for imagining an HIV/AIDS otherwise, whether there is a different way of navigating HIV/AIDS in the world within our vastly heterogeneous but often inequitable systems of care.

Put another way: Who is "the end of AIDS" (working) for? Who does the discourse serve, and to what uses will it be put? For whom is AIDS to be ending? And what is at stake when the process for bringing about HIV/AIDS' end practically relies on the disease's chronicity in at least three ways: as experienced over the course of an individual life of managing a lifetime on therapies whose long-term effects into old age remain understudied; as a collective experience among PLHIV and their kin who are managing stigma, treatment, and aging into chronic HIV infections; and as experienced through and practiced in administrative time (i.e., the funding and implementation cycles for HIV programming, which will likely be separate from care, as long as this agenda is the agenda). I limit this reflection to a handful of chapters in this book, as I am myself grappling with the possibility of the end of AIDS and looking to my colleagues' rich ethnographic material for guidance and insights.

Practically, this means asking (and answering) whether testing is accessible and desirable for people living in the sites in question; who pays for testing, care, and drugs and for how long; how do drugs "get into" bodies and suppress viral loads? and what other forms of solidarity, attention, and support will be needed to ensure strict adherence to treatment regimens among the populations most vulnerable for the foreseeable future? These are all complicated matters that also impel us to use HIV/AIDS as a prism through which we examine relations of power, ethics, and health, as our authors show us through discrete case studies of people living with HIV/AIDS across the globe.

The virus and the syndrome it causes draws its symbolic strength from and warps in its favor the markets shaping health policies and practices; from a clinical and ethical perspective, it renders notions of care and caregiving semi-intelligible, casting light on itself as the rightful object of care; and from a technical perspective, it may create inequitable bureaucratic practices and norms. The "end of AIDS," therefore, is at once a political tool, an ethical ideal, and a public health goalpost, in that any allegiance or fidelity to this message will require careful consideration of how resources materialize, are managed and distributed across steeply graded inequalities specific to the regions where this agenda is operationalized in a manner aligned with justice and equity. Will reaching the benchmarks be sufficient to end AIDS and its social, political, economic, and bodily sequelae? How will "ends" and the interventions that bring them about be experienced, felt, and lived through? Answering these questions requires reckoning with systemic and steeply graded inequalities operating across different spatiotemporal scales. In the US South, where I was born and raised—and where much of my family resides—the progress toward this goal has been stymied by generalized decrease in social safety nets, health infrastructure, and financing. In Sierra Leone, where I studied the institutions that provide care, support, and treatment for PLHIV, it became clear that providing supports that exceed and extend beyond an HIV diagnosis or HIV-specific categories of vulnerability would require significant reordering of donor-recipient relations at the national levels, of agenda-setting beyond goals set elsewhere (Benton 2015).

Space-time relations via a discourse of "the end of AIDS" become compressed or confused with each other, amplifying rifts and inequalities the places that serve as the sites of study here. For whom can HIV/AIDS end when there is no cure; for whom can HIV/AIDS end if the disease is imagined to be "chronic"; for whom can HIV/AIDS end if chronicity is the means and the goal? As Murray has reminded us in his introduction to this book, we are now in the fourth decade and close to starting a fifth decade of a "global pandemic" in many parts of the world: How does the "long durée" of a disease (which apparently is not nearly as long as the handful of diseases we have effectively eliminated or eradicated from entire regions), coupled with "compressed" end of crisis discourses and their resultant practices, impact HIV/AIDS policies and protocols? How does it affect the lives of people living with HIV?

Walsh Lang writes about the experiences of children and their NGO-based caregivers in a Ugandan HIV treatment residential facility for HIV+ children. This research raises important questions about how regimes of care developed in an era of effective HIV therapies, shape ideas about family and kin networks of care. Specifically, the author presents an interesting paradox: While children's HIV status is either downplayed or abstracted from discussions about their well-being, their status as well as their families' ability to manage the illness shapes whether these children can be successfully "reintegrated" into their families and communities. I could not help but be struck by the resonances between this program and, say, drug rehabilitation programs, as well as postwar demobilization and reintegration efforts that took hold in the 2000s throughout Latin America and sub-Saharan Africa. For evaluating the stakes of AIDS' "ends," we might consider what these experiences tell us, what is at stake in removing, "reeducating," rehabilitating, and reintegrating children to better "cope" with their HIV status, as a way of preparing them—and their kin, many of whom are also HIV+—for a lifetime on medications, an adolescence of constant surveillance and assessment. These children arrive at the center in crisis: Gender and kin relations appear to be interrelated with the (re)production and management of HIV stigma; under these circumstances, who can imagine the end of AIDS, and what would such imagination engender for thinking kin with stigma over the life course?

Through Hassan's careful rendering, we learn about how HIV becomes a political tool through which Egyptian innovation, state-sanctioned moralities, and national rebuilding are configured and mediated. Specifically, a device invented for the purpose of detecting and curing hepatitis C and HIV, and the clinical trials to test the device's efficacy, become both a case study for Hassan to investigate the aforementioned process of HIV's politicization, and an opportunity for the state to invest in projects of dubious efficacy, for the (cynical?) sake of consolidating an appearance of state efficacy via its technological innovations and biomedical in(ter)ventions. Hassan's chapter explores this through an "exorbitant analogism" (Seltzer 1995), in which the body politic and individual bodies are thought together, with the Egyptian military asserting its role in clinical experimental regimes, and the extension of military metaphors into narratives about the disease and state attempts to diagnose and cure comorbidities of concern. The language comparing the immune system to the military offers confirmation of what we might have intuited: Metaphors of military organization and armed struggle continue to organize perceptions of HIV/AIDS—even in the decades since Sontag (1989) wrote about AIDS as metaphor inflected by violence and threats posed by "others" and Emily Martin (1990, 1992) elucidated vernacular and expert renderings of the immune system's defensiveness. In my own work with the Sierra Leone military's HIV/AIDS unit in the early 2000s, the deep entanglement between state agents of violence and order, and disease management pose a conundrum for those who envisioned a biopolitics articulated in terms of care and support (Benton 2015). The case described by Hassan, however, affords the reader an opportunity to think of the stakes of "the end of AIDS," when the body politic and HIV+ Egyptian women's bodies are coextensive with each other—the extent to which political transformations via and after the revolution lend special resonance or relevance to the invention and legitimization of this set of technologies and a global agenda of AIDS' end. Put another way, the fantasy of cure becomes intertwined with the national(ist) fantasies and desires that coalesce around concepts like innovation and achievement and is fulfilled through an "end of AIDS" agenda. What, then, does attention to Egyptian state practices and political context offer us, as we decipher this global agenda, its legitimacy and its consequences for people living with HIV/AIDS in Egypt?

Ordóñez, drawing on extensive ethnographic research in South Africa, compellingly shows how global biomedical and local neoliberal models of care have struggled to sustainably manage the antiretroviral therapy program in South Africa due to, among other key political and economic factors, a lack of recognition and acceptance of the strong plurality characterizing the health-seeking behaviors of HIV patients and the implications of this situation for the effectiveness of the health care system. The chapter hones our focus on an important question: How does a global HIV agenda, ordered around particular norms of care-seeking, distort or occlude visions of care that lie outside globalized models that both imagine a narrow view of care's enactments and reflect a bias toward biomedicine (and toward biomedicine as antiretrovirals and norms of adherence)? In arguing for recognition of medical plurality and the variations in therapeutic itineraries navigated locally, Ordóñez is also critiquing a faith in "standardization" and normalization that does not account for actually existing care (and health) modalities. I was particularly struck by the potential for "alliance" versus partnership or integration, particularly if we are to think of "partnership" as a kind of folk model of global health that formalizes relationships of inequality through bureaucratic and administrative means. Again, the chapter brings us to an earlier question: Who is "the end of AIDS" for? Whom does it—as a discourse, as a political tool, as a goalpost—serve?

Finally, I turn to Thiongane and Graham's careful study of an Ebola vaccine clinical trial among PLHIV in a West African site, which was initially argued to be "a reflection on temporality and locality of being HIV positive enough to participate in an Ebola vaccine trial." It is perhaps more importantly an account of how HIV distorts and mediates "standards, normality and location; treatment, cure and prevention; and colonial inequities, race and power." The benefits of the clinical trial and participation in it are largely dictated on biological markers of HIV positivity, and the social and biological qualities that are presumed to accrue to adhering to certain norms of positive living. The chapter pursues a number of paths and paradoxes that I was forced to reckon with, as a scholar who has studied the social worlds constituted through and around both HIV and Ebola in West Africa. We have a reason to be hopeful: there is promise of efficacious vaccines, treatments, and cures for Ebola. And there is hope that all of these will be available to people living with HIV/AIDS. Participation in the trials for each of these clinical interventions renders the paradoxes of "positive living" visible: The "chronic" status of their HIV illness requires lifelong commitment to consuming therapies that may very well limit their ability to participate in the trials for HIV+ people. In other words, they qualify for the trials because of their HIV status, but they may be excluded from participation if their therapies work too well, or as intended; or they might be excluded if these therapies do not work well at all.

Together, these chapters compel us—from the bottom up, and across scales—to think about what a global agenda to end AIDS might look like from the perspective of PLHIV and to ask for whom will AIDS "end"? For whom does "the end of AIDS" obtain meaning? On whose terms? Through which means, and at what cost, will this end be achieved? What could this kind of ambitious goal-setting make possible, if subtended by a radical vision of health and well-being? We have to imagine an otherwise.

REFERENCES

Benton, Adia. 2015. *HIV Exceptionalism: Development through Disease in Sierra Leone*. Minneapolis: University of Minnesota Press.

Martin, Emily. 1990. "Toward an Anthropology of Immunology: The Body as Nation State." *Medical Anthropology Quarterly*, 4, no. 4 (December): 410–26.

Martin, Emily. 1992. "The End of the Body?" *American Ethnologist* 19(1): 121–40.

Seltzer, Mark. 1995. "Serial Killers (II): The Pathological Public Sphere." *Critical Inquiry* 22(1): 122–49.

Sontag, Susan. 2001. *Illness as Metaphor and AIDS and its Metaphors*. New York: Macmillan.

Index

Note: *Italicized* pages refer to figures/tables and page numbers followed by "n" denote endnotes.

About the Editor

David A. B. Murray is professor of anthropology and sexuality studies at York University, Toronto. He is the author of *Opacity: Gender, Sexuality, Race and the Problem of Identity in Martinique* (2002), *Flaming Souls: Homosexuality, Homophobia and Social Change in Barbados* (2012), and *Real Queer? Sexual Orientation and Gender Identity Refugees in the Canadian Refugee Apparatus* (2015). He is the editor of *Homophobias: Lust and Loathing Across Time and Space* (2009) and *Queering Borders: Language, Sexuality and Migration* (2016).

About the Contributors

Adia Benton is an associate professor of anthropology and African studies at Northwestern University, where she is affiliated with the Science in Human Culture Program. She is the author of the award-winning book, *HIV Exceptionalism: Development through Disease in Sierra Leone*, and is currently writing a book about the 2014–2016 West African Ebola outbreak.

Janice Graham is a medical anthropologist, professor of pediatrics (infectious diseases), and University Research Professor at Dalhousie University. She has been studying regulatory practices in the development of emerging therapeutics and vaccines in Canada, Europe, and Africa for over 25 years, focusing on safety, efficacy, and trustworthiness in the construction and legitimization of evidence. Graham is particularly interested in transparency, open data, public health, and the commercialization of publicly funded innovations. She is a fellow of the Royal Society of Canada.

Wesam Hassan is an anthropologist and a physician. Currently, she is a PhD candidate in social anthropology at the University of Oxford, in which she is working on state-regulated games of chance practices and perceptions. Prior to her academic career, Wesam has worked with the United Nations and international NGOs in public health and population issues with a special focus on HIV and AIDS, harm reduction, and sexual and reproductive health and rights. Since 2016, she has been researching material culture and consumption habits by conducting and analyzing several ethnographies in Iran, Egypt, London, and Turkey. These ethnographies have investigated womanhood and cleaning rituals in Iran, online gambling and betting in London, and the perception and usage of the Internet of Things and smart homes as a concept in Egypt.

Jallicia Jolly is a writer, postdoctoral fellow and incoming assistant professor in American studies and Black studies at Amherst College. Dr. Jolly researches and teaches on Black women's health and activism, reproductive justice and health inequities, and intersectionality and HIV/AIDS in the United States and Caribbean. She is working on her first book manuscript, *Ill Erotics: Black Caribbean Women and Self-Making in the Time of HIV/AIDS*, an ethnographic and oral history study of the erotic lives and grassroots mobilization of young Black Jamaican women living and loving with HIV/AIDS while building empowerment, navigating structural oppression, and contesting pathologizing discourses of HIV containment. Dr. Jolly's scholarship and community-engaged work foregrounds the interrelationship between lived experience, pedagogy, and political engagement and fosters a black diasporic feminist agenda in the Americas and the African diaspora. Her work has been supported by grants and fellowships such as The Fulbright Scholar Program, The Mellon Mays Foundation, Yale University's Sarah Pettit Fellowship, Brown University's Pembroke Center for Teaching and Research on Women, and the National Women's Studies Association.

Robert Lorway is professor of medical anthropology in the Institute for Global Public Health, University of Manitoba, where he holds the Canada Research Chair in Global Intervention Politics and Social Transformation. His research analyzes how forms of intervention and life unfurl around transnationally mediated attempts to alleviate the suffering of stigmatized people. He has written two books on the subject, *Namibia's Rainbow Project: Gay Rights in an African Nation* and *AIDS Activism, Science and Community across Three Continents*.

Claudia E. Ordóñez, anthropologist and MA in intercultural relations, is adjunct assistant professor in the Hubert Department of Global Health at the Rollins School of Public Health of Emory University. Using the lenses of medical and applied anthropology, her research interests include HIV/AIDS, plural health systems, and traditional African medicine with a focus on community-engaged research approaches, interdisciplinary and transdisciplinary research collaborations, and intercultural proficiency conceptualization, evaluation, and training. She teaches courses in Community Health and Development at Emory University and maintains a flourishing set of ongoing biomedical and public health research collaborations with colleagues in South Africa and in the United States. She is proudly a Colombian immigrant.

Pamela Runestad earned her PhD in anthropology at the University of Hawaii at Manoa and is currently an assistant professor of global health studies at Allegheny College in Pennsylvania. Trained as a medical anthropologist and Japan specialist, she has research interests in infectious disease, food and health, and Asian societies. Runestad's forthcoming book, Vulnerable Bodies: Living with HIV in Japan, is part of the medical anthropology series on health, inequality and social justice at Rutgers University Press.

Vaibhav Saria is an assistant professor in the Department of Gender, Sexuality, and Women's Studies at Simon Fraser University. They are the author of *Hijras, Lovers, Brothers: Surviving Sex and Poverty in Rural India*, published by Fordham University Press.

Stephen L. Schensul, PhD, is professor emeritus of public health sciences at the University of Connecticut, School of Medicine. He received his BA in anthropology from Hunter College of the City University of New York and his MA and PhD degrees in anthropology from the University of Minnesota. He learned applied anthropology and participatory research in the formation and development of health and mental health programs in collaboration with activists in the Chicano neighborhoods on the west side of Chicago and continued this work in Miami and Hartford, Connecticut, over the next two decades. For the past three decades, Dr. Schensul has focused on HIV and prevention of sexual risk in Mauritius, Sri Lanka, India, and Vietnam with funding from the US National Institutes of Health. He is the recipient of the Career Award from the Society for Medical Anthropology; the University of Connecticut Provost's Faculty Award for Excellence in Public Engagement and shares the Kimball Award from the American Anthropological Association for Public and Applied Anthropology with Jean J. Schensul.

Oumy Thiongane is a medical anthropologist (CIRAD-UMR Astre: Animal Santé Territoire Risques Ecosystèmes) and research associate at Dalhousie University (Technoscience, Regulation and Research Unit). She leads extensive work on epidemics and vaccines in West Africa and has conducted several ethnographies in biomedical laboratories. Recently, she has worked on data science and technologies in European surveillance systems, with a particular interest in how modeling informs COVID-19 decision making in France and Finland. She also is leading a new study on the ethical issues of digital health in the surveillance of infectious diseases.

Colleen Walsh Lang is a resident physician in Emergency Medicine at Loma Linda University Health in Loma Linda, California (USA). She graduated from the combined MD/PhD program, at Washington University in St. Louis (USA) in 2020 with her degree in anthropology. Her dissertation was titled *Vulnerable Agents: Ugandan Children's Experiences with HIV Rehabilitation and Reintegration*. Additionally, Colleen completed a fellowship in clinical medical ethics at the MacLean Center for Medical Ethics at the University of Chicago (USA) in 2018–2019, and currently, she serves on the ethics committee at Loma Linda University Medical Center. In 2010, Colleen founded a small nonprofit organization to provide additional support to the organizations she works with in Uganda. In her spare time, Colleen enjoys walks in the neighboring hills with her "pack"—her husband, son, and dog.

www.ingramcontent.com/pod-product-compliance
Ingram Content Group UK Ltd.
Pitfield, Milton Keynes, MK11 3LW, UK
UKHW020840290926
15470UKWH00004B/1462

9 781666 901481